Inspiration

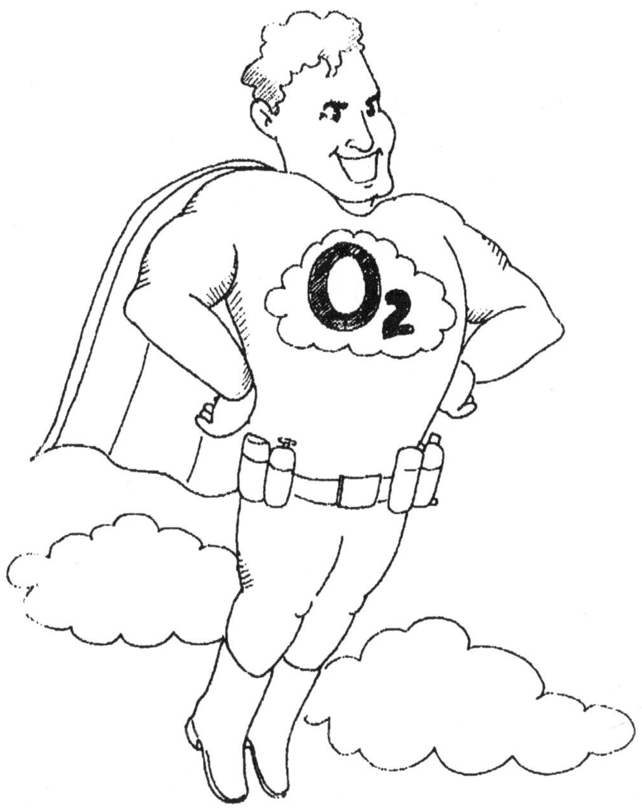

Your guide to better breathing

by Margaret A. Varnell, RN, RRT

Illustrations by Brian Lazar

FOWLER & WELLS

PUBLISHERS

Originally Established 1836

Good Communications, Inc.

PO Box 10069, Austin, TX 78766

(800) 968-1738

Inspiration

Your Guide to Better Breathing

by Margaret A. Varnell, RN, RRT

ISBN: 0-937776-11-4
Published by Fowler & Wells, Publishers
An imprint of Good Communications, Inc.
PO Box 10069, Austin, TX 78766
(800) 968-1738 E-mail: gooddogmag@aol.com
Additional copies of this book are available at a group discount, or booksellers discount. Please contact Good Communications, Inc. at (800) 968-1738 for prices.

Publisher: Ross Becker
Managing Editor: Judith Becker
Assistant Editor: Amanda Braziel

Printed in the United States of America
First Edition: October, 1998

About The Author

Margaret A. Varnell is a Registered Nurse and Registered Respiratory Therapist. She successfully completed the NBRC's Perinatal Pediatric Specialty Board in 1992. She is a former Director of Pulmonary Rehabilitation and works as a consultant throughout the U.S., Central America and the United Kingdom establishing Breathing for Stress Reduction, Asthma Management, Inpatient and Outpatient Pulmonary Rehabilitation Programs, Smoking Cessation Programs, and as an advisor to Pulmonary Medicine Services. She has more than 400 articles in print in various medical journals and was the recipient of The Bird Award for outstanding medical reporting in 1996. She is a field correspondent for *Advance for Respiratory Care Practitioners*. She is the Allied Health Delegate to the Information Delivery Committee for the American College of Chest Physicians, a member of the American Association of Respiratory Care, and a member of the American Medical Writer's Association. She is also a regular contributor to *Sneeze The Day!,* the newsletter for people with allergies and asthma.

Miss Varnell is also known for her work with WYES-TV Channel 12 in New Orleans, where she has written and produced numerous shows including: Yellow Jack: A History of Yellow Fever; Angels in New Orleans; A 50th Celebration of *A Street Car Named Desire*; Haunter of Ruins; Pretty Baby; and others. She is presently working on a new series about Louisiana artists entitled, *By Louisiana Hands*. She is the Editor of *Impressions*, the newsletter of the International Edgar Degas Foundation and is a member of the Board of Directors of the Shakespeare Festival at Tulane (for which she directs the Swan Series).

Contents

Introduction

Best while you have it use your breath,
There is no drinking after death.
John Fletcher

Breathing is one of the most-studied of all human endeavors. The Vedas of ancient India, written more than 4000 years ago, extol the proper practices and techniques of breathing. Breathing exercises form the foundation of many meditative traditions, including yoga and Tai Chi. They're said to be a window to the soul, a key to harmony and balance, and a portal to a deeper understanding of yourself.

Breathing is also one of the most forgotten and overlooked of bodily functions. Most of us don't think much about it until we don't do it so well. Then we think a lot about it and we want the problem fixed fast.

I have had the privilege of helping many people "fix" their breathing problems. Whether you are a corporate executive learning to control your stress, an actor learning to better use your voice, a mother about to deliver twins, a COPD patient, or a smoker trying to quit and deal with the changes in your body, the basics are the same. You need to know how your breathing works and how you can make it work better for you.

This book is designed to do just that. It is a basic overview of how your breathing works. Most importantly, this book will help you understand what's going on with your breathing in simple, plain language, so you can talk to your doctor about it. Breathing is an integral part of life. You deserve the knowledge that helps you make informed decisions about it. Here it is.

Margaret A. Varnell
New Orleans, Louisiana
October, 1998

Full of sweet dreams and health, and quiet breathing.
John Keats

Part 1
The Basics

Breathing 101

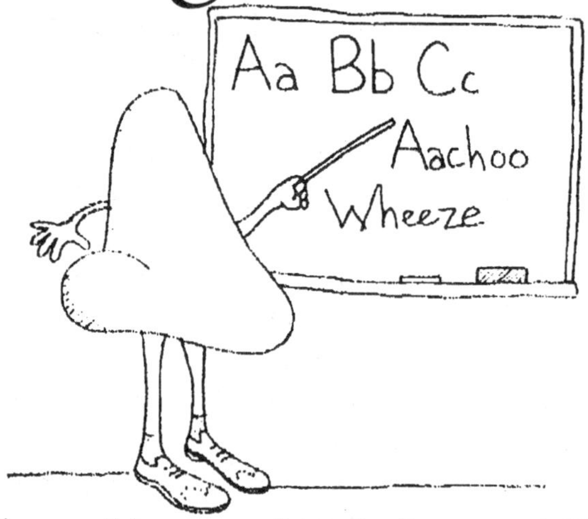

Breathing is something most of us take for granted. The unconscious flow of air moving in and out of your lungs provides the needed oxygen for your body and carries away the used gases.

Yogis and wise men from the East have spent centuries studying the process. They say that your breath can bring you closer to God. Scientists and physicians the world over have studied the mechanism and devoted millions of dollars to unlocking the keys to our breathing. Still, much of this vital process remains a mystery. Let's look at what we do know about how your breathing works.

The Basics of Breathing

Air flows into your body via the nose or mouth. Inside the nose there are structures called the nares. The inside and back of the nose is called the nasopharynx. Above and behind the nose are large, empty cavities – the sinuses. The air flows past these cavities onto the oropharynx, which is the back of the mouth. Your nose is the first filter system, warming the air you breathe, adding moisture or humidity, and screening out the large dust and dirt particles. You can't see much of what goes on inside your nose, but, you can locate the oropharynx.

The easiest way to see your oropharynx is to look in a mirror and open your mouth. In the back of your throat you'll see the uvula, a pink, tear-shaped structure hanging down. That area at the back of your mouth is your oropharynx. When you're breathing through your mouth, the air bypasses the nose and flows directly into this space.

There are two possible paths air can take as it flows through the oropharynx. It can go down the windpipe, or trachea, which carries air to the lungs. The alternative is the food pipe, or esophagus, which usually carries food to the stomach.

The epiglottis is a flap of skin that closes over the trachea to protect you from food going down into your lungs. It looks kind of like a Frisbee® and closes off the windpipe when you contract your throat to swallow. Occasionally, air is swallowed and goes into the stomach. This won't hurt you – it'll come back out as a burp or as flatulence.

When food gets misdirected into the airway, the body responds by coughing to expel it. We all know what that feels like. Coughing is the body's defense mechanism for expelling unwanted debris from the airway.

The larynx, or voicebox, is just inside the trachea below the epiglottis. This is where the vocal cords live. The larynx isn't essential to breathing, but is necessary for talking. It can become infected and swell, closing off the trachea and making breathing difficult. Still, the larynx has no actual role in the breathing process.

The trachea branches off into smaller pipes as you go deeper into the chest. The first branch occurs at a junction called the carina. Here the pipe splits into the right mainstem bronchus and left mainstem bronchus, which carry the air either to your right or left lung. The trachea and right and left bronchi are often called the central airways. Their purpose is to carry large quantities of air to the airways below. These central airways are made up of donut-like rings of cartilage. Between these donuts are muscles called bronchial smooth muscles. These are the muscles that constrict and cause asthma sufferers so much trouble.

From The Outside

Let's step outside for a breath of air and look at your chest. From the exterior, your chest looks the same on both sides. What you can't see is that the right and left lungs are a little different from one another. What they do is the same, and functionally, their internal structure is the same, but their external structure is a little different. The right lung has three lobes or segments. This means that on the right side of your chest the mainstem bronchus must split into three areas. The left lung only has two lobes or segments, so the main bronchus only has to split into two areas. The reason for this difference in your two lungs is very simple, when you remember that your heart takes up the space in the left side of your chest where the third segment would be.

Now gently place your hand on your stomach and slide it up. Do you feel the "stop" or point where your abdomen stops and your chest starts? That's the diaphragm. It's the main muscle of breathing.

Place your hand back on your stomach and breathe in deeply. Feel your chest expand? That's because you subconsciously told your diaphragm to pull down on your chest. The air flowed in to fill the space in your lungs when your diaphragm pulled down or flattened out. As you exhale, your diaphragm pushes back up and the air is pushed out. You told your diaphragm to do all this work via the vagus nerve.

The muscles between your ribs, the intercostals, help the diaphragm. When you're having difficulty breathing, these muscles work very hard to help out. This can easily be seen in babies. When a mother sees her child working hard to breathe, she sees the muscles pulling on the baby's ribs. These are called retractions. This is one of the first signs mothers of asthmatic babies are taught to look for. Adults can have them too, but they are more difficult to detect.

Back Inside

Now that we've looked at the outside, let's go back inside and see where the air is going. Back in the airway, the pipe has split into the right and left sides. It will continue to split further as it travels deeper into the chest. Along the way, the smooth muscles are gradually replaced by a different type of wall structure. The new walls are made of various types of cells. There are goblet cells that secrete a thick mucus, as well as other cells that have different jobs.

The walls of the lower pipes have more layers of cells as you go deeper. The top layer has a lining of very fine hairs called cilia. The cilia are like the shag carpet of the lungs. They wave back and forth rhythmically, to a beat. The cilia do this because sometimes particles and debris get to the lower airways. The movement of the cilia is the body's way of moving the debris up and out to a point where it can be coughed up and expelled. If you've been to a rock concert and seen someone picked up by the crowd and moved along overhead, then you know what the ciliary action looks like.

Mucus secreted in the lower airways has many functions. The very thick mucus catches the debris particles and moves them along. Thin mucus acts as a lubricant for the lungs.

All in all, the airways bifurcate, or split, about 25 times before the air finally gets where it is going. At the bottom of the last airway branch are the alveoli. These are little grape-like sacks where respiration occurs.

Ventilation and Respiration

Let's talk a minute about some of the finer points of words. Up until now we have talked about air moving in and out. This is called ventilation. It's where most asthmatics have their problem. They can't move the air in because their central airways tighten up. Instead of breathing through a wide pipe, they are trying to move air through a straw.

In contrast, respiration is the actual movement of oxygen through the alveoli of the lungs into the blood. It's important that you understand the difference between the two terms. Air has to move in and out (ventilation) for it to be picked up by the bloodstream (respiration). But simply moving the air in and out doesn't mean that oxygen will go into the body. You see, ventilation can occur without respiration.

The difference between ventilation and respiration is the defining difference in most airway disease. We can treat either ventilation problems or respiration problems. Sometimes we only have to treat one, and sometimes we have to treat both. But the mechanisms and drugs available to treat these two conditions are different.

Inside The Alveoli

Let's go back inside to the alveoli. As we said, this is where the oxygen from the air you breathe crosses into the bloodstream. Carbon dioxide, the body's principal waste product, also moves out of the blood via the alveoli.

As you can imagine, the alveoli are pretty busy. Yet the blood doesn't actually enter the alveoli. Instead, the blood streams by in the capillaries, like cars on an Interstate highway. The oxygen must merge, and the carbon dioxide exit. This generally occurs without a mishap. The oxygen is picked up by the hemoglobin of the red blood cells and taken along for the ride.

When the hemoglobin has all the oxygen it can carry it's a bright red color. This can be seen from outside the body as a pink, rosy color to your skin. When the hemoglobin can't pick up the oxygen, it's a bluish color. This can also be seen through the skin. On cold days, when your hands get cold and your fingernails turn blue, it just means that the hemoglobin, weighed down with oxygen, can't quite get through to your fingertips. So you rub your hands together to warm them up. As the oxygen-charged blood flows again to the extremities, they pink up. This "turning blue" phenomena is called cyanosis. It can be harmless, like on cold days, or it can be a sign of either a ventilation or a respiration problem and can be very serious.

Several conditions can stop the respiration process from occurring. Sometimes the grape-like alveoli will collapse, especially if they haven't been used in a few breaths. This is called atelectasis. The alveoli look like balloons that have not been blown up.

Atelectasis actually happens several times a day. Your body corrects the problem by taking in a big breath and reinflating the sacks. This is usually what's happening when you sigh or yawn. In babies whose alveoli, or air sacks, have never been blown up, it's a bigger issue. Lower airways becoming clogged with mucus can also cause atelectasis. The air can't get to the sacks and they collapse. Cystic fibrosis patients have unusually thick mucus that does this. If you have asthma or allergies, this may occur when you have a cold or are dehydrated. COPD patients can have atalectasis and mucus – sometimes at the same time.

Those are the basics of breathing. Specific illnesses and conditions have their own peculiarities and circumstances, but everyone's lungs work the same way.

How your lungs work

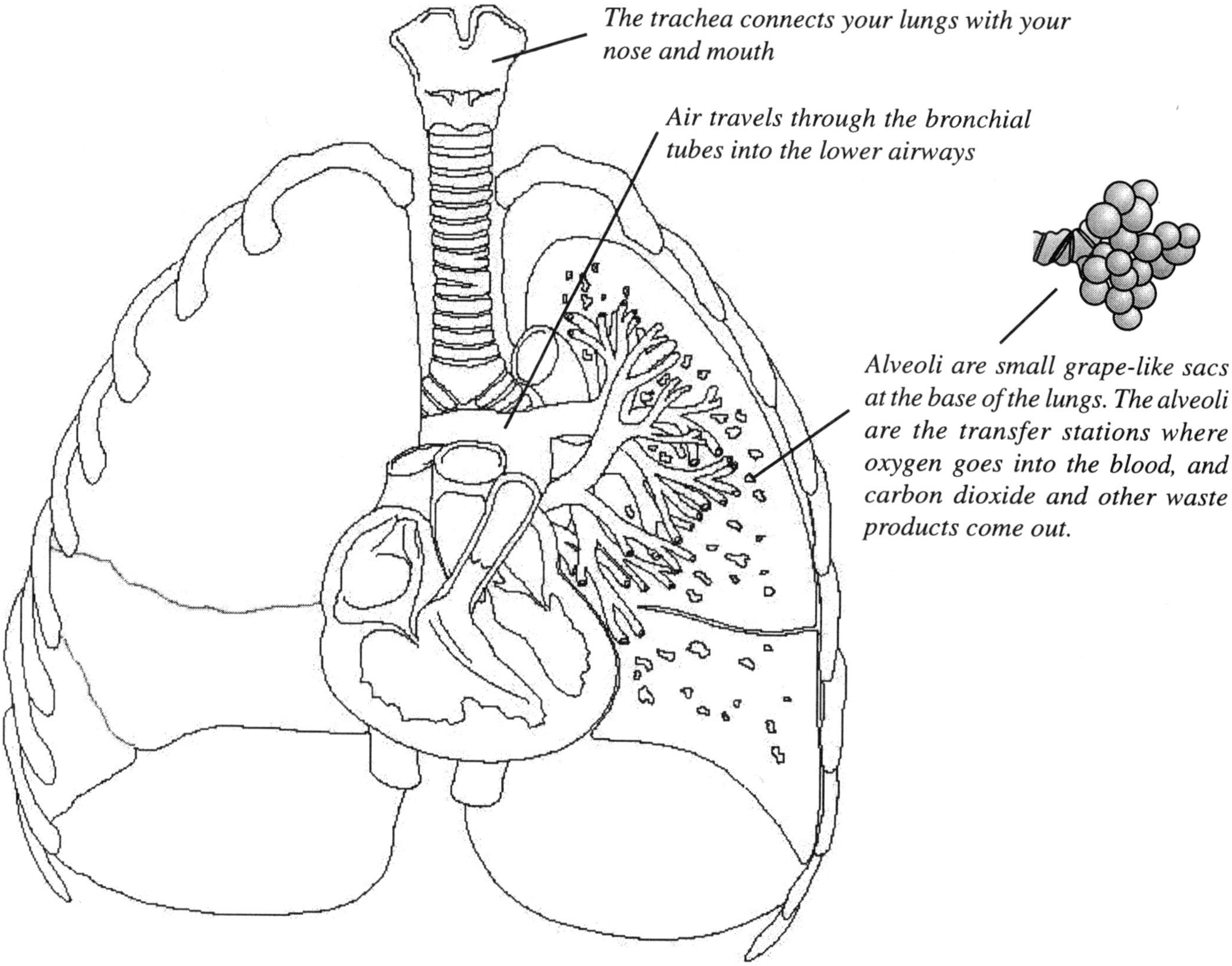

How your immune system works (or doesn't)

Your body is a wondrous thing. Its structure and design is pure genius, undoubtedly wrought by a higher power. Who else could have designed such elegant complexity? The further scientists delve into the workings of the body, the more amazed they are at the sophisticated mechanisms they find.

One of the most exciting areas of medical research is immunology, the study of the immune system. Because of all of the money devoted to HIV/AIDS and cancer research, new developments are being announced daily. The world's understanding of the functioning of the immune system grows each year, and new medications are being developed to take advantage of the new knowledge.

But what is the immune system? How does it work? And why does it sometimes go haywire, resulting in allergies and asthma? Why are new therapies trying to circumvent or interrupt the immune response? These are all basic questions immunologists are trying to answer. And the answers are the keys needed to solve the problems of allergies, asthma, and other inflammatory diseases. Here are some basics.

The body has many ways of protecting itself against invaders. The skin keeps the vast majority of nasties outside, and the good stuff inside. Sneezing and coughing expel foreign gunk as it tries to enter the nose or lungs. There are many antimicrobial (mostly antibacterial) secretions in skin and mucous surfaces, which add another level of protection. The acidity of the stomach (a pH of 0.9 to 1.5), and the mucus and upwardly-beating cilia of the bronchia help kill and push out other invaders.

Still, some clever foreign substances make it into the bloodstream. They're generally dealt with by the immune system. The immune system has the responsibility of recognizing when bacteria or foreign substances enter your body. First it sounds the alarm and lets the rest of the body know that the invader has arrived, so the troops can be rallied. Then, it battles with the invader.

We all have some inborn mechanisms which fight certain bad guys. This is called *natural resistance.*

How Vaccines Work

The *adaptive immune response* creates antibodies which specifically fight each type of invader. After the microorganism is killed off and you recover from the illness, your body is sometimes left with *specific memory,* which enables the body to quickly deal with the same microorganism if it returns. This is called *acquired resistance.* (A vaccination presents an inactivated or harmless version of a microorganism, which stimulates the body to create resistance to the dangerous version of that microorganism.)

Since the body doesn't know what's going to be harmful and what's not, it

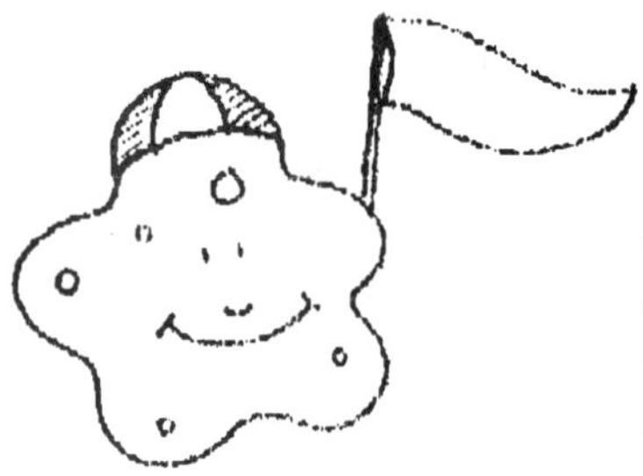

Stem cells travel to the thymus and become T-lymphocytes, which fight infection. They can also become phagocytes – the trash collectors of the immune system – or T-helper cells, which alert the body to invading germs.

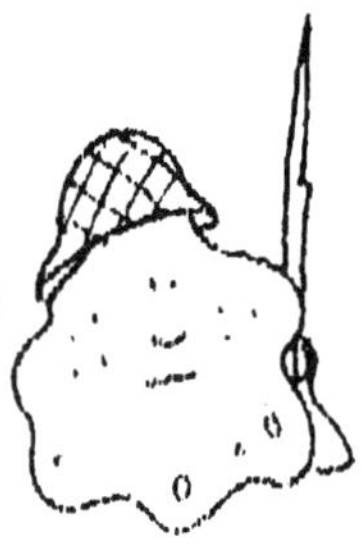

T-Lymphocyte – the infection fighter

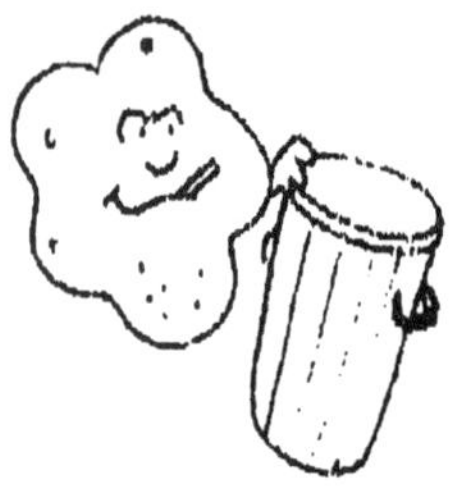

Phagocytes are the garbage collectors

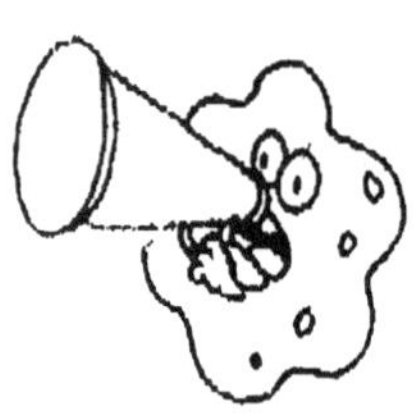

T-helper cells call in assistance

responds to all foreign material as though it were harmful. That can include harmless things like pollen. Pollen gets the same immune response as, say the flu bug. But when the pollen returns next year, the specific memory may cause your body to react even more strongly, with *hypersensitivity,* and all of our favorite allergy symptoms.

Your immune system is tailored to your needs and has been modified by your experiences. Your body produces antibodies specifically for each invader, as well as for pseudo-invaders in vaccines. So my immune system is going to contain different antibodies than yours, and will offer me faster protection against the invaders my body is already prepared to fight against.

Here's how it works. Your immune system screens every single particle that enters your body. It identifies those which are good for you, like oxygen, and lets them pass without incident.

It also has to recognize the particles that are normal and naturally produced by our body. These are called *self* substances. *Non-self* substances are the bacteria, viruses, fungi, and toxins that enter your body and can cause damage or illness.

Another name for a non-self substance is an *antigen* or *allergen*. These are of particular interest to the immune system, as they are the things the body must respond to.

Since each body's immune response is slightly different, what is a normal self substance to one may be a non-self substance to another, and vice versa. For example, ragweed may be considered an irritating substance by your body, but not by mine.

Autoimmune Disorders

When your body gets the self and the non-self substances confused, you're said to have an *autoimmune disorder.* Your body does battle with the self substances instead of the non-self substances that it should be focused on. There's a great deal of research going on right now that is trying to identify asthma and allergies as autoimmune disorders.

Autoimmune disorders (which include lupus) are different from immunosuppressive disorders. In autoimmune disorders, the body fights against itself, confusing good and bad. In immunosuppressive disorders such as HIV, the immune system becomes overwhelmed by the virus and its functioning is suppressed. While HIV and asthma are very different, both involve the immune system. Researchers in both fields are sharing knowledge, and expanding their understanding of the immune system.

A Normal Immune System

Let's get back to the basics. The immune system is made up of organs and tissues in the body, specifically the thymus gland, the liver, spleen, lymph nodes, bone marrow and blood.

The bone marrow is the first area we'll examine. Marrow is the fleshy, center part of your bones. It's critical because its main job is to make blood cells. Even more important is that the marrow is also the factory where baby immune cells are made. These cells are called *stem cells*. They are basic, generic immune cells that have the ability to develop into a lot of different types of mature cells.

Stem cells are like high school graduates who haven't decided on their career yet. There are three career choices for stem cells. They can become B lymphocytes (B cells because they're derived from bone marrow), T lymphocytes (T cells because they're derived from the thymus), or phagocytes.

B lymphocytes or B cells turn into plasma cells in our blood. The plasma cells go on to make immunoglobulin. That's what most of us call antibodies.

Antibodies

Your body can produce antibodies to millions of different substances. A good way to think of the B cell/antibody connection is to consider the B cells to be the temp workers of the immune system. They go into the bloodstream and hang around until a job becomes available. When a particular type of antibody is needed, they become that type, and go to work. These antibodies are one of five classes: IgG, IgA, IgE, IgM, and IgD.

IgA is found in all secretions of the body. It's the major antibody in the mucous membrane lining the intestines, and in the saliva, bronchi (in the lungs), urine and tears. IgA blocks microorganisms which have made it to these external surfaces, keeping them from getting into the tissues themselves. IgA then triggers an antigen-antibody reaction.

IgD is a specialized antibody. It appears to work only on the surface of B cells. It increases in quantity during allergic reactions to milk, penicillin, insulin and certain toxins.

IgE provides the primary defense against allergens in the environment. It's concentrated in the lungs, the skin, and the cells of mucous membranes. IgE is the antibody which causes those big red skin reactions. IgE is a particularly hot topic of research among asthma medication manufacturers right now.

IgG responds to bacteria, fungi, and certain viruses. It can gain access to the fetus through the placenta. There are many subclasses of IgG, each of which responds to a different antigen.

IgM is usually the first type of antibody made in a response. It's also thought to have been the first antibody to appear during evolution. It's very effective at tying up and destroying microorganisms.

T Cells

The white collar workers of the immune system are the T lymphocytes or T cells. The college they're bound for is the thymus. The thymus is an organ located in the upper center part of your chest. Here, the stem cells grow up. There are three types of T cells that they can become.

The first type of T cell is the T lymphocyte or the soldier cell. This is the one which goes out and actually fights the invaders.

The second type of T cell is the T helper cell. These are the cells that marshal the troops. When an invader enters the body, the T helper calls the B cells and tells them what type of antibody to make. They also help the T lymphocyte cells know when and where the battle will be.

The third type of T cell is the T suppressor cell. These are the cells that call off the battle. Basically, they keep a running tally of the battle and how it's going. When it's over, they call the B cells and tell them to slow down production. They step in and calm down those younger T lymphocyte fighter cells that are chomping to get into the action.

Phagocytes

Phagocytes are the next type of battle cell that a stem cell can become. These are relatively quiet cells. They are the trash collectors of the immune system. The *free circulating phagocytes*, including *leukocytes,* float around in the blood and eat anything that is not supposed to be there. The word phagocyte, in fact, means "cell-eating." Their principal diet is microorganisms like bacteria or viruses. Once they eat, they digest their meal by creating a chemical which kills the microorganism. The good thing about phagocytes is that they can leave the bloodstream and travel through the tissue of the body to eat microorganisms. They aren't terribly particular about where they find their meals.

Macrophages or MACs, are another type of phagocyte. They're large tissue cells responsible for eating damaged tissue, cells, and bacteria. While part of the natural immune system, MACs also have an important role to play in setting off the adaptive immune system.

The Complement System

The *complement system* is the last component of the immune system that we'll take a look at. Basically the complement system is a family of eighteen different blood enzymes which help out the phagocytes and produce widespread inflammatory effects. Some are made in the liver, others are made by the phagocytes.

The complement system makes the overall adaptive immune system run more smoothly. Some of the enzymes attach themselves to a microorganism like a big flag and make it easier for the immune system to see it. Other complement functions include coating the microorganism and making it easier for the phagocyte to swallow.

There are a few other players in the immune system that we haven't mentioned. The liver makes a lot of the complement system proteins. It's also phagocyte central. Some of the phagocytes that prefer not to float around in the blood set up housekeeping in the liver and wait for the blood to come to them. There they filter the blood and eat any microorganisms that come along.

The spleen is another organ that plays a key role in the immune system. It's located just behind the liver, sort of an exclusive suburb of the liver. Many of the T cells and B cells prefer to live in the spleen, waiting until they're called out to battle.

Finally, there are the lymph nodes. These are located all over the body. They are like regional T cell and B cell police stations, filled with defenders waiting for something to happen. When an invader microorganism does move into their neighborhood, the lymph node springs to life. The local B cells begin making antibodies, the T helper cells sound the alarm and the town quickly becomes flooded with out-of-town T and B cells ready for the fight. This massing of defenders is what causes your lymph nodes to swell.

Now you know the basic elements of the immune system.

Immune System Disorders

How do you know if you have an immune system disorder? Most of these disorders are generally recognized while you're still a child. That's because you'll get many infections, and they'll keep recurring.

Usually these infections occur in the sinuses or the chest, but you may also have frequent bouts with diarrhea. This is caused by an overgrowth of the normal bacteria found in the digestive tract. Basically, the immune system can't keep the normal bacteria's numbers under control.

There are tests which can assist your doctor in identifying immune system problems. For the most part they're blood tests. They measure the different numbers and types of immune system cells that are in your blood system. Sometimes, more advanced bone marrow testing may be necessary.

What do you do if you or your child is diagnosed with an immune system disorder? The first thing is not to panic. Millions live normal, healthy lives and are scarcely impacted by the illness. Minor life-style adjustments and increased awareness of how their bodies work is all they need. People with a depressed immune system should eat right, get plenty of rest and exercise, and be aware of good hygiene techniques to prevent the invasion of the nasties. Things like washing hands before you eat, after going to the bathroom, and after shaking hands with someone become even more important than normal. The National Immune Deficiency Foundation is also a good source of material and educational assistance. They can be reached at 1-800-296-4433 or write: The National Immune Deficiency Foundation, Courthouse Square, 3565 Ellicott Mills Drive, Unit B2, Ellicott City, MD 21043.

For most of us with allergies, the problem is the opposite – an overimaginative immune system. When the immune system is activated with adaptive responses, inflammation results. When this becomes a nuisance, it's hypersensitivity.

Immunosuppressants like corticosteroids (cortisone) can temporarily interrupt or suppress the immune response, allowing things to calm down. (They also open up the body to invasion, since the immune system is being put on hold.) Antihistamines and other drugs can interrupt certain stages of the immune response, and reduce inflammation. Immunotherapy (allergy shots) is supposed to re-educate the immune system so that antigens don't cause a wild response.

Since you can reduce, but not eliminate, exposure to the antigens that bug you, drug therapy is the alternative.

Scientists are learning more about the detailed workings of the immune system and of each antigen. As they do that, they find new ways to "tie up" the invaders and prevent them from reaching the immune system targets which stimulate the immune response. That means new and better drugs to help those of us with out-of-whack immune systems.

References

Janeway, CA, Travers, P. ImmunoBiology: The Immune System in Health and Disease. Second Edition, 1996. Current Biology Ltd.

Playfair, JHL. Immunology at a Glance. 6th Ed., 1996. Blackwell Science

Buckley RH. Immunodeficiency Diseases. *JAMA* 258:2841, 1987

Primary Immunodeficiency Diseases: Report of a World Health Organization Scientific Group. *Immunodef Rev* 3: 19, 1992

Patient and Family Handbook for the Primary Immune Deficiency Diseases, Immune Deficiency Foundation. 1993

Allergic Diseases Diagnosis and Management, Patterson, Roy, MD (editor) 4th edition, J.B. Lippencott and Company, 1993

COPD, a family of breathing illnesses

Lung disease is, unfortunately, a fact of life for millions of Americans. Sadly, most don't have the opportunity to sit down and have their particular conditions explained to them. Making things even more confusing is an abundance of terms. You've always been told you have asthma, but now they say you have emphysema, but all the books they give you are for COPD. Well, let's clear the air a little bit and see if we can get all this straight.

COPD

Chronic Obstructive Pulmonary Disease (COPD) is a catch-all term for a family of diseases. It simply means that for some reason the air flow into and out of your lungs is obstructed or blocked. This obstruction can be caused by inflammation, tightening, or collapse of the airways. Depending on the cause, one of two things may happen: air becomes trapped in your lungs and gets stale; or you have difficulty getting air into and out of your lungs, and you have to work harder to breathe. In most cases, a little bit of both occurs and you feel short of breath. Let's take a specific look at some of the illnesses that are grouped under the COPD umbrella.

Emphysema

Emphysema is a disease that occurs in the very bottom of your lungs. The little grape-like sacks in your lungs (alveoli) begin to stiffen up and enlarge. Normally, these sacks expand when you breathe in and then contract a little when you breathe out. This contraction helps to push the air up and out of your lungs. In emphysema, however, they expand and don't contract. That means the air stays in and gets trapped.

Your body gradually attempts to adjust to this expansion and your diaphragm becomes pushed down and flattened. To breathe, you must now work this muscle even harder. Most emphysema patients learn to compensate by using their shoulder muscles to breathe. For many, the most comfortable position for breathing is leaning slightly forward, with arms propped up in front on a shoulder-height table.

Smoking is the most common cause of emphysema, though heredity, pollution, and occupational factors can also contribute to the condition.

Pulmonary Fibrosis

Pulmonary Fibrosis is a condition in which fibrotic material, similar to scar tissue, forms in the airways. It can form at the alveolar level or in the air pipes themselves. It usually occurs after infections or a prolonged illness. It is difficult for individuals with this condition to breathe because they can't get air in easily. In addition, the lung area where the oxygen goes in and the carbon dioxide comes out is usually blocked by the scar tissue.

Bronchiectasis

Bronchiectasis is the next airway illness we'll take a look at. It's a structural dysfunction of the bronchial tubes. Basically, it's a condition in which the bronchial tubes, or the lower breathing pipes, become distended and stay that way. It can occur as an injury after an infection or it can be an abnormal development from birth. Most patients notice that they cough a great deal when they change positions. This is because the damaged pipes don't move the lung secretions very well, and it takes moving to shake the secretions up and get them on their way up and out of the lungs. It's very easy for bronchiectasis patients to contract frequent infections if they're not vigilant about coughing regularly and keeping the secretions moving out of their lungs. This condition is often confused with chronic bronchitis.

Chronic Bronchitis

Chronic Bronchitis occurs when the lining of the airway becomes irritated and responds by producing extra secretions. These extra secretions are an ideal environment for bacteria to grow in, helping infections to occur. They also clog up the airways and make it harder for the individual to breathe. Regular bronchitis occurs once and the individual recovers from it. For the condition to be considered Chronic Bronchitis, it must last for three months and occur each year for a minimum of two years.

Asthma

Asthma is both an inflammatory and a restrictive disease. In other words, the airway is irritated, so it produces extra mucus to flush out the irritation. Then, it contracts or squeezes because it's irritated. The squeezing of the airways, or spasms, coupled with the excess mucus clogging things up, are what make it difficult for you to breathe during an asthma attack.

Allergies

Allergies are a reactive disease. They are reactive because, when something irritates your airway, your body responds by flooding the area with excess secretions. This is what causes runny noses. Allergies are not traditionally a part of the COPD family, but because they are so closely linked to asthma, I'm mentioning them here as a "cousin by marriage."

Clubbing

Clubbing of the digits is not an illness. It is a sign. It is a change in the angle of the nail bed that occurs as a result of chronic illness. We don't know exactly what causes the change, but it can occur in either your fingers or your toes or both. It is not dangerous. It's just a change that occurs over time, which your physician may notice and comment about.

These are the basic illnesses that make up the COPD family. It's not unusual to have more than one, or mild versions of a few of these illnesses.

Three treatment approaches are applied in varying degrees to all of these conditions. If an infection occurs, we use antibiotics and good coughing and hygiene techniques to clear it up. If the airway is inflamed, we try to use medication to reverse or stop the inflammation. If the airway is narrowed, we use a medication to widen or dilate it. The specific medications you use will depend on your specific needs at the time. Your doctor, pharmacist and healthcare provider should take the time to discuss what you're taking as well as your specific illness.

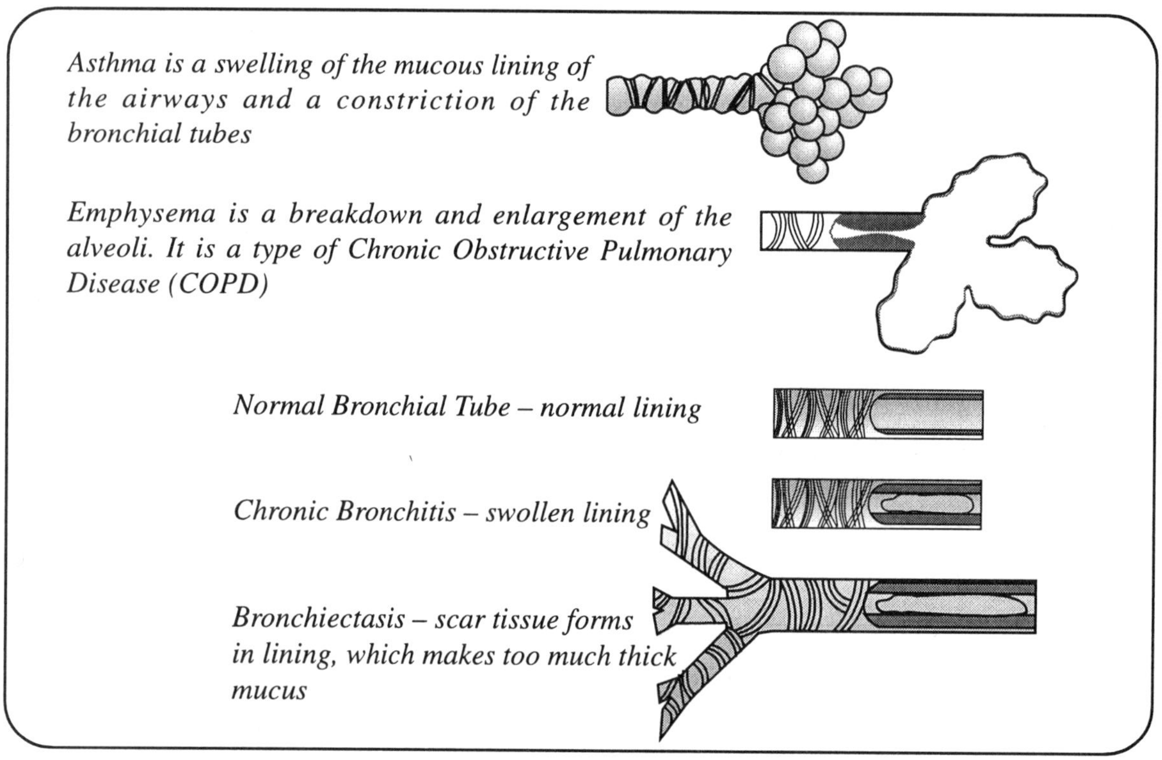

Everything you need to know about health tests

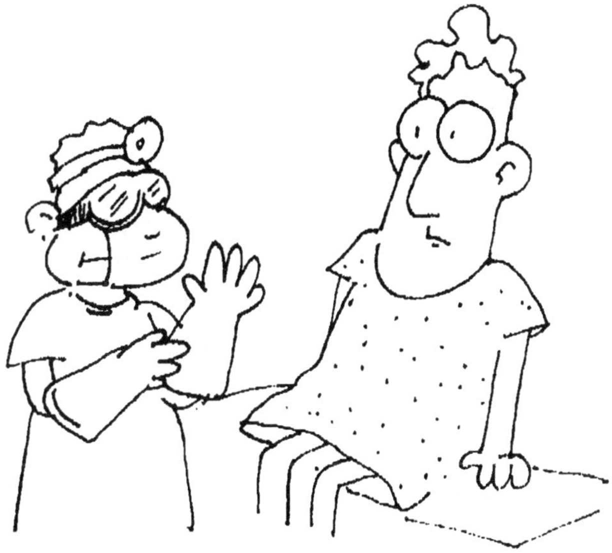

You're sick, and the doctors can't figure out what's going on. Is it allergies? Or something else? Tests are ordered to get more information. Health tests are some of the best ways to gather information about your body. They're a wealth of information to the person who understands them and can interpret the data.

As a pulmonary patient, your doctor will give you the usual barrage of blood work and urine studies, plus some tests specific to your condition. If you have other, mysterious health problems, you'll get deeper into the testing process. Let's look at each test, why it's given, and what it can tell about your health.

If you're experiencing a life-threatening illness and require immediate medical attention, your doctor may alter the sequence of testing based on your immediate needs. Sooner or later, though, he should come back and complete the tests he omitted.

Medical History

Let's first look at the basics. The most important source of clues your doctor relies on is *you*. So, the first thing your doctor will do is collect as full and complete a medical history as possible.

He'll begin by asking a lot of questions. This can be annoying and may not seem relevant. But chances are these questions and your answers will help him establish a clear picture of who you are and what your life is like.

For asthma,allergy or COPD patients, this is crucial. The doctor is trying to identify the triggers that cause your allergic reactions. It's important that the findings be both subjective (what you think), and objective (what the lab and test results show).

Let's say allergy testing suggests you're only allergic to dog dander. But the reality is you have no problem being around your Golden Retriever, it's just when the neighbors' cat comes to call that you become congested. Then, obviously the lab tests aren't telling the complete story. Only you can fill in the gaps.

The questions will be about your home, office, pastimes – pretty much any activity or environment that's part of your daily life will be subject to scrutiny. As the history progresses, your doctor will begin narrowing the field of inquiry in the hope of identifying a specific antigen (substance) that triggers your body's allergic response.

The Physical

Once your oral history is taken, the doctor will begin your physical examination. In addition to the usual vital signs of blood pressure, pulse, respiratory rate and temperature, your doctor will be looking for specific physical symptoms caused by your illness. Your eyes, throat, sinuses, ears, chest and skin will all be examined for clues.

A common allergic response of the eyes is conjunctivitis. This is a swelling of the membranes of the eyes. To you, it's that itchy, watery, weepy feeling. To your doctor, it's hyperemia and edema – clear indicators that something's irritating you. In severe cases, it can show up as a bluish discoloration. You and I call it dark circles under the eyes.

Rhinitis (a runny nose) is what the doctor looks for next. Careful attention should be paid both inside and outside your nose. No, this isn't pleasant (think how *he* feels!), but your doctor should look up your nose and down your throat.

If your sinuses are so congested that there's drainage going down into the back of your throat (the dreaded postnasal drip), your doctor should start you on the appropriate medication to control it. He should also note whether your sinuses are puffy or tender, and thus full of congestion.

Perhaps the most disgusting thing he'll do will actually be easy for you: he should look at your sinus drainage. This means you'll have to blow your nose for him. He'll note the color, the thickness and if there's any smell coming from your drainage. All these symptoms could be indicators that there's something going on besides your allergies.

The rule of thumb on sinus drainage is: If it's clear or white, it's okay. If it's yellow, green or discolored, there's probably an infection going on. If it's pink, there's obviously bleeding somewhere.

Next, the doctor will examine your ears. He'll look in them and possibly even swab them with a Q-Tip® to see if there's any infection in there.

Your Chest

Moving away from your head, your doctor will examine your chest. He'll probably listen to your heart, but his main concern will be evaluating your respiratory status. He'll note if your breathing is easy or labored, and if it's symmetrical. In medical jargon, this is referred to as your work of breathing.

If you favor one side of your lungs over the other, there's probably a reason. Your doctor will need to delve deeper. That means you should be auscultated. Now, don't panic! That just means listening to your chest with a stethoscope. He'll listen to the way the air moves into and out of your chest. This can tell him a lot.

If you have asthma, the bronchial rings of your trachea contract. It's difficult moving air through that narrowed tube. This creates a raspy or wheezing sound. It occurs in asthma, emphysema, and in acute allergic situations. Whether the wheezing is caused by asthma or a major allergic response, it needs immediate medical attention.

If congestion and inflammation are filling up your chest, this can also be heard with the stethoscope. It sounds like a gurgling or rattling noise made as the air passes through the secretions. To your doctor, it sounds like water boiling. The fancy terms for this are rales or crackles.

Your Skin

The next thing your physician should look at is your skin. Your overall color is important. Are you flushed and red as if you had a fever? Or are you pale and bluish? Cyanosis is a bluish discoloration caused by a lack of oxygen in the blood. We all know how our hands look when we're very cold. And how our lips can turn blue from the cold. That's an environmentally-induced cyanosis. This condition can occur if there's something going wrong inside your body, as well.

Darker-skinned people won't turn the traditional blue; instead, they'll have a grayish or ashen tint. The doctor should be on the lookout for this, and he should evaluate your overall appearance. Most likely, he'll look at your nail beds in the process. This is a rule-of-thumb indicator of both your pulmonary and your cardiac status. Are they pink and healthy, or are they blue? When pinched, how quickly does the blood return? This is called the capillary refill time. A normal capillary refill time should be almost immediate. Your doctor will note this.

Clubbing is a condition that occurs with many chronic pulmonary diseases. We don't know specifically why it happens, but we do know that it's an indication of persistent hypoxemia or low blood oxygen levels. It's simply a swelling of the base of the nail bed that changes the angle of the fingernail. It's very difficult to diagnose in the early stages, and almost impossible if the doctor hasn't seen you before. It's difficult to tell what's normal and what's abnormal for you without a prior reference point. Still, most doctors will make a note of it as part of their evaluation.

Swelling

Your doctor will also look for specific signs of edema or swelling. Specifically, he or she will be looking for pedal edema,which is swelling of the ankles. This gives an overall idea of how your kidneys and – indirectly – how your heart are working. The doctor may also listen to your stomach to make sure it growls. This is his way of verifying that your digestive tract is on track.

A Closer Look At Your Skin

In the final part of the physical exam, your doctor should examine your skin. If you're allergic, you may suffer from a histamine response in the form of a rash. You may also have atopic dermatitis – an allergic response through the skin. You may not necessarily call it a rash, though, because it can take on many different forms.

Medically speaking, it begins with erythema, or redness. This may develop into a papular rash, which looks a bit like a diaper rash. These papules can become blister-like. They're called vesicles when they take this form. The blisters can pop, ooze and be quite uncomfortable.

Usually, people are seen in various stages of this process. They may have erythema in one spot, and oozing vesicles in another, simultaneously. A bacterial infection would love to set up housekeeping in these lesions, so the oozing vesicles should be kept as clean and dry as possible.

If you have a long-term case of atopic dermatitis, lichenification of the skin occurs. The skin becomes hard, red or discolored, and raised. It may also be very dry and scaly, and, it can be itchy, too. Think of it as allergic scar tissue.

Pruritus, or itching, is perhaps one of the most subjective symptoms a patient can have. There's no hard and fast rule as to when you will itch and when you won't. It could occur at any phase in the process and it's different for each person. But the itching is very real and should be taken seriously by your doctor.

Deciding What's Next

After your physician takes a complete medical history from you, and after he has conducted a thorough examination, he should sit down with you and discuss his preliminary findings. At this time, further lab tests and possible diagnosis should be discussed. Your doctor should be willing and able to explain any testing he wishes to pursue, and why. If he's not willing to do this, find another doctor. And, if after looking at you this closely, he can't at least map out a path for you to take, chances are he's not up-to-date on how to deal with allergies and asthma. You deserve someone who is.

Lab Tests

Most testing is done by independent pathology laboratories, although bigger medical centers have their own in-house laboratories. Results come back as a computer printout, with your results in one column, and a normal range printed next to it for comparison.

While lab tests are often expensive, and frequently used to cover the behinds of doctors, they're also the quickest and easiest way to zero in on a problem. Here's our guide to understanding what each test is, and what it can tell you:

Arterial Blood Gases (ABG). The Arterial Blood Gases test is frequently ordered by doctors. It uses blood taken from an artery, blood that's carried away from your heart and taken to the tissues of your body. Testing this blood is useful because it has just come from the lungs. It's important to examine the components of arterial blood to see, not only how your heart and lungs are functioning, but what your body tissue has to work with in terms of oxygen. This blood test can also give physicians some insight into how your kidneys are functioning.

To fully understand this test, let's review a little about how your body works. Your lungs are your body's main source for getting oxygen into its system They're also a primary way of getting rid of waste products like carbon dioxide (CO_2). Your kidneys are another way the body filters blood and gets rid of waste products. There's a delicate balance between the pulmonary (lung) and the renal (kidney) systems. If one has a bad day, the other can pick up some of the slack and keep your body going.

An ABG measures the level of waste products in your blood. Because it's blood that's coming directly from your heart and lungs, it's a more exact measure of lung function. But, indirectly, the elements of the kidneys' job can be seen. In fact, the three questions your physician wants the ABG to answer are: Is your body taking in oxygen? Is your body getting CO_2 out of itself? And, is there a proper balance between your kidneys and lungs?

The first value reported is the pH. This is a measure of the acid/base balance in your body. If you have too many waste products, you're acidic and your pH is lower than normal. If, for some reason, your body has eliminated too many of the waste products and upset the balance, then your pH rises and you're alkalotic. A normal pH is around 7.40.

PaO_2,or the partial pressure of oxygen in the arterial blood, is the next number reported. This is a measure of the amount of oxygen that the hemoglobin is carrying around to the tissues of your body. In other words, it shows how much oxygen is being absorbed into the bloodstream. A normal value is 80 to 100 mm Hg. Ideally, this means that most of the hemoglobin is carrying oxygen (the remainder is resting and waiting to carry oxygen in an emergency).

PCO_2, or the partial pressure of carbon dioxide, is the next value shown in the ABG report. This is a measure of the carbon dioxide that's in your blood. As we mentioned before, this tells your doctor if that all-important balance of waste products to good substances is being maintained. Remember, this is primarily a measure of how your lungs are keeping up their end of the bargain. A normal PCO_2 is 35 to 40 mm Hg.

To keep an acid in balance we must have a base. The base in the body is bicarbonate. It's represented on the report as H_2CO_3. A normal bicarb value is 22 to 26 mEq/L.

Base Excess or BE is the fifth value reported. This is a calculated number that's done at the time the blood is analyzed. It's an estimate of how much of the waste product or good products would have to be added to the blood to bring the pH and PCO_2 to their normal values. For your body, this shows how much work the kidneys are going to have to do to keep the balance. A normal BE is approximately 0, plus or minus 2.

Blood and Urine Tests

Why do doctors want blood and urine samples? Most people don't mind donating these bodily fluids to Medical Science. But few understand the tests and what the results mean. Let's take a look at some common lab tests and what the resulting numbers tell us.

The reason for lab work is twofold. Either your doctor is trying to get a measure of your overall health, or wants to see if you're responding to a medication. If your body is fighting an infection, your lab work will reveal how the struggle is going, and whether or not an antibiotic is or isn't helping. Depending on the type of lab studies performed, the tests may also point to the specific antibiotics that will work to battle the infection.

Complete Blood Count

The most common blood test ordered is a Complete Blood Count or CBC. A small amount of blood is taken, and the laboratory literally counts the number and types of cells in the sample. The number of each variety of cells is reported and compared to other types of cells. These figures help determine your health status.

Red blood cells (RBC) are also known as erythrocytes. The RBC is a count of these cells. These cells are very important to the proper functioning of the body because they carry oxygen. If you have pulmonary problems, the level of RBCs is an indicator of your lung condition.

RBCs are looked at from two perspectives. Laboratories use these two perspectives to report two different numbers to the physician. **Hemoglobin** is the part of the RBC that carries oxygen around. Iron is a principal component of hemoglobin. If your body's iron level is low, you're anemic. This means your body can't produce the hemoglobin it needs to carry the oxygen around.

The other way laboratories look at your RBCs is by reporting your **Hematocrit**. This is a measure of the number of RBCs in your blood. It's reported as a percentage of your total blood values. This balance of RBCs and other blood components lets your doctor know how you're doing, overall.

Many pulmonary patients have difficulty getting oxygen into their blood. Since the body wants to take advantage of every possible oxygen molecule it can get, it makes more RBCs. This is known as polycythemia. It doesn't occur in every pulmonary illness, but it can be a good indicator of a chronic or ongoing problem, and it's a big, red flag for your doctor.

If you're completely confused, let's stop and look at RBCs another way. Think of your blood as a highway system that moves around your body. The RBCs are the buses, and the oxygen represents the passengers. The hemoglobin is the number of seats on the buses. These seats are made up of iron. So, when they measure the hemoglobin, they're measuring the number of seats available on the buses. The Hematocrit is a count of the total number of buses.

White blood cells are the next blood component which laboratories like to count. White blood cells are also known as leukocytes. Their principle job is to fight off infections and keep us healthy.

There are many different types of white blood cells and each has a different job as part of the body's defense system. The laboratory counts these different types of white blood cells and also calculates the percentages of each. This is called a WBC with differential.

Fluctuations in the types of white blood cells can tell a lot about what your immune system is struggling to overcome. Allergy sufferers often have an increase in eosinophils. Higher levels of neutrophils can occur in cases of infection and severe stress. Lymphocytes are another type of white blood cell that often become elevated in response to viral infections. Various other types of white blood cells can help pinpoint if you have a viral or a bacterial infection.

Let's use an analogy to make this clearer. Think of a highway (the bloodstream). There are plenty of vehicles on the highway (red and white blood cells). The white blood cells are emergency vehicles on patrol in your body. There are a certain number of police cars, ambulances, and fire trucks on routine patrol at any given time. If a bacterial infection (a fire) breaks out, your body responds by sending all available fire trucks (neutrophils) to the site. All available police cars (leukocytes) also respond and try to help out. As the fire continues, the body responds by making more fire trucks and police cars to help out. So the number of neutrophils and lymphocytes in the blood rises. This increase is shown in the laboratory report and tells your doctor that there is, indeed, a fire going on.

A **Complete Blood Count** (CBC) could be called the traffic update of your body. It's a measure of the red blood cells and their components, Hemoglobin and Hematocrit, and the white blood cells and their components. It lets your doctor know whether everything is running smoothly, or if there's a small snarl (infection) that's growing into a major jam that's making you sick.

More stuff in your blood

We've taken a look at blood cells. Now let's look at other frequently-performed lab tests and see what *they* mean. **Platelets** are an important part of our body's defense mechanism. Smaller than blood cells, platelets can be thought of as our body's internal Band-Aids®. When an injury occurs, the platelets rush to the site and clump together. A normal value is 150,000 x 350,000 mm^3. Many illnesses can cause fluctuations in your platelet level. The measure most often seen is a **Prothrombin Time/Partial Thromboplastin Time** or PT/PTT. This measures time it takes your body to form a clot in response to an injury.

Glucose is another name for sugar. A normal fasting value is 70-110 mg/100 ml. The pancreas helps the body regulate the blood glucose levels by producing a hormone called insulin. A low level of blood glucose levels is known as hypoglycemia. A high level is known as hyperglycemia.

Cholesterol is a lipoprotein. It can be taken in with the food you eat, and it's also naturally produced by your liver. There have been many reports of good and bad cholesterol, and differences in opinion as to what a safe blood level is. The prevailing thought today is that a result of 200 mg/dl and below is still considered acceptable for adults.

There are many different types of cholesterol. **High Density Lipoproteins** (HDL) is good cholesterol. **Low Density Lipoproteins** (LDL) is bad cholesterol. **Triglycerides** are another type of cholesterol – the unknown cholesterol. There are no definite studies linking elevated triglycerides as a risk factor for coronary artery disease, but there are no studies definitively excusing them, either.

The **Serum Drug Levels Test** is a measure of the specific blood level of certain drugs. The most common of these is a **serum theophylline** level. Blood is taken and measured to see if the level of medication available in your blood is enough to handle your problem, or if you need more to regulate your illness. The ideal level is 10-20 micrograms /milliliter.

Urine Tests

A **Urine analysis** is a common test. Basically, the lab takes a look at the cells they find suspended in your urine. The specific gravity or density of the urine is reported. The color, odor, and pH are reported, as well as whether or not certain cells are present.

In a urinalysis, the lab looks for levels of glucose, blood, and bacteria in your urine. Creatinin levels are also checked. This is a measure of kidney function. It's most often reported along with a blood test of the patient's **Blood Urea Nitrogen** level or BUN. These two measurements help give a more complete picture of the functioning of your renal (kidney) system.

Fecal, Sputum, and Throat Tests

Fecal tests are becoming more common. They're inexpensive and can often be done in the doctor's office. They usually test for blood in your stool. This is a screening test for colorectal cancer, polyps and other conditions that can cause bleeding in your lower digestive tract.

Doctors often request **Sputum cultures**. This is an examination of the mucus in your lungs. The sample is obtained by asking you to cough something up. The laboratory places some mucus on a growth medium and attempts to culture the organisms that are currently in your sputum. The bacteria that's infecting your lungs is what they're looking for. If they can isolate the specific bacteria, then they can recommend the most potent antibiotic for treatment. This is the most definitive way of identifying the bacteria that cause illness. A problem with this test is that it doesn't offer immediate results, and it can't be used to identify viruses, only bacteria.

A **Throat culture** is similar to a sputum culture. The difference lies in the collection process. For a throat culture, a long swab is used to wipe the back of the throat and collect a sample for the laboratory to culture. In babies and children, a nasal swab may be done rather than a throat swab. The laboratory then tries to grow and identify the offending bacteria.

EKG, Pulse Oximetry, X-rays

Your doctor might also request a host of physical tests. An **Electrocardiogram** (EKG) is a test that looks at the electrical activity of your heart. The heart is the muscle that pumps blood throughout your body. It does this by squeezing or contracting and pushing the blood into the blood vessels. An intricate series of electrical impulses tell the different parts of your heart when to contract and when to relax. The EKG measures these impulses and how fast they're going. If they run into a roadblock – so to speak – they have to detour and go another way. Your EKG will show this. So, in this way, your doctor can take a look at how your heart is operating.

Pulse oximetry is a harmless test that can performed anywhere. It's a measure of the amount of saturated hemoglobin circulating in your blood. Because the hemoglobin usually carries oxygen, it's indirectly a measure of how much oxygen is available in your blood for your body to use. The nice thing about this test is that it's done without taking blood. It works by putting a probe or clip on your finger. One side of the probe sends out a red light that goes through your finger and measures the amount of light that passes through your finger. Some of the light is deflected by the blood as it passes through, and some of it passes through undisturbed. The oximeter then uses the measured data to calculate the saturated level of hemoglobin in your blood. This test is quick, painless, and inexpensive.

X-rays are still a commonly-used tool. A chest X-ray is perhaps the most likely screening test your doctor will order. Basically, X-rays take an electromagnetic picture of your body. The rays pass through soft tissue, but not hard tissue. Bones show up as bright and white. Cartilage, which is less dense and softer than bone, shows up as ghostly white or gray. The rest of the tissues show up as black because the X-rays pass completely through them.

If you have pneumonia or fluid in your lungs, it will show up on your chest X-ray as an area that's more white than it should be. Other conditions can also be diagnosed from X-rays, thereby assisting your doctor in establishing a clear, overall picture of your health status. The main reason for taking an X-ray is to rule out an infection or some other disease process that may be going on.

Sinus X-rays can be useful for chronic allergy sufferers. They don't really assist the doctor in diagnosing the allergy as much as they give a picture of what's *not* wrong. Because many allergy sufferers experience frequent sinus infections, a series of X-rays can determine if there is something structural contributing to the infections. Is there a hidden pocket that affords a safe harbor for bacteria to grow? Or are there are any changes in the sinuses that commonly occur in allergy sufferers. (These are usually a *result*, not a cause of the allergy.)

Tests for the Allergic

There are some tests that are specifically used for allergy sufferers. These tests help your physician develop a complete picture of what's going on inside. Specifically, they're trying to identify what triggers your allergic response and how to respond to it. To do this, they intentionally expose you to the offending allergen in a small dose to see what your response is.

Skin tests are the most common. These tests require preparation and discussion before use. In particular, you should be free of allergic symptoms and your skin should be clean, healthy and intact. If you have a rash, it's best to postpone the test, as conflicting results could occur and the test would have to be repeated.

You also can't take any antihistamines and antibiotics for at least two days before the test. And there are some medications that require a longer time to flush out of your body; you must stop taking these for a longer time. Your physician should discuss and explain all this to you.

There are two types of skin tests approved for use in the United States: the **prick test** and the **intracutaneous test**. The prick test consists of pricking the skin with a needle that has been contaminated with the allergic antigen solution. Allergic antigen solution is a fancy way of saying it's a standardized extract of the thing your physician thinks you're allergic to.

This test is typically done in the doctor's office. Several rows of antigen drops are usually placed on your arm and then each drop is pricked. A clean needle should be used with each prick and, if a prick draws blood, the test for that particular antigen should be repeated.

The good news is that the tests can be read within 30 minutes and there is rarely an anaphylactic (shock) reaction. Of course, you may be shocked by the results!

The bad news is the test isn't very sensitive and the accuracy, when compared to intracutaneous testing, is not as good.

The intracutaneous test involves injecting a small amount of the allergic antigen into the outer layers of the skin. This method is more accurate because the antigen is actually placed inside the body and the body responds. But the very fact that your body is responding adds an element of risk. Your body can have a really small reaction, or a really big reaction.

A prick test prior to an intracutaneous test is a good idea. In this way, the doctor can be more specific in the types and numbers of antigens he or she uses in the intracutaneous test. The doctor is able to rule out the multitude of allergens that you didn't respond to at all and not use them in the intracutaneous test.

In educated, skilled hands, this is a very safe procedure. A reaction will occur within twenty minutes of injection if you're allergic to the antigen. To be safe, you should be monitored throughout the process.

Delayed reactions can occur, but usually do so within 2 hours. If you're going to have a reaction, it will most likely be in the form of a big, red wheal or welt. Your doctor will measure the size and redness of the welt, and also note any other changes you may be experiencing, such as itching.

If you leave the doctor's office and have a delayed reaction to your test, notify your doctor at once. You probably aren't in any danger, but the reaction must be graded within a certain time frame or the test won't be valid.

The Passive Transfer test is not used here in the U.S. The best way to explain this is to compare it to the "rabbit test" of old. A serum collected from an allergic person is injected much like in the intracutaneous testing procedure. Only it's injected into a non-allergic person. The non-allergic person is then "challenged" with an injection of the antigen at the same site. The health risk to the non-allergic test subject is certainly obvious in this day of communicable diseases. But this test is still on the books and is also known as Prausnitz-Kustner Testing.

Provocation testing is another form of challenge testing. You are intentionally given an antigen (allergy-causing substance) to see how your body responds. Introducing an antigen to someone's eyes or nose is possible, but terribly uncomfortable and usually unnecessary. Skin testing can demonstrate the allergy without making you miserable.

Bronchial Provocation testing for asthmatics is more common. This is the process of making a spray (aerosolizing) out of an antigen and having you breathe it in. An asthma attack should then occur. In most cases, this is a last resort in the diagnosis of asthma. Other means can be employed to document your illness.

Histamine release and IgE screening are blood tests that may be used in the future. Histamine release testing is useful in research studies and may have a clinical application in the future. But to date, nothing that really helps the ordinary allergy sufferer has been developed.

IgE screening, however, is a different story. Through a complex series of laboratory procedures, we're able to isolate whether or not you're sensitive to a particular antigen. The problem is that there's no universally accepted standard for the level of positive reaction. There have been studies comparing it to skin testing and about the only honest answer anyone can give is that both have their good points and bad. The decision to use either should be discussed with your physician.

Dietary challenges are growing in popularity. A specific food is omitted from the diet and the response is gauged. Later, the food is added back to the diet, and the response is again gauged. There are some who swear by this technique. But from a medical point of view, it's difficult to quantify and measure the results. For food allergies, though, it's still considered the most reliable way of determining whether you'll have an allergic response after *eating* a food.

The **ALCAT Test** is a blood test for food and chemical hypersensitivities which is quite accurate, although not very well-known. Your blood sample is challenged with the different foods and chemicals, and a special blood analyzer measures very subtle changes in the size and count of white blood cells. The test must be performed within 28 hours of the blood sample being taken, and only one lab in the U.S. is equipped to perform the test (although the blood can be drawn anywhere).

Pulmonary Function Tests

Pulmonary Function testing is frequently ordered to assist your doctor in evaluating your lung status. This is a series of tests that measures the volumes of air you're able to move into and out of your lungs, the speed at which you're able to move that air, and what your lungs do with that air while it's inside.

People with known or suspected pulmonary disease are frequently asked to complete pulmonary function tests. Allergy sufferers, as a rule, are not, but they may encounter the tests as part of a preoperative screening. These tests are frequently given prior to surgery so the anesthesiologist can determine lung function.

The most common pulmonary function study – and one done at home every day by millions of asthmatics and COPD patients – is the **peak flow measurement**. This is a forced exhalation through a hand-held device that reports a number value. The number is a reflection of how open and relaxed your airway is.

A **Negative Inspiratory Flow** is occasionally performed. It's a relatively simple procedure. Basically, the peak flow measures how hard you can blow out. This test measures how hard you can pull a breath in. It's unlikely that an asthmatic will be asked to do this.

Spirometry is the most basic pulmonary function test done in the office or hospital. It's inexpensive and relatively simple. You're asked to take in a deep breath and exhale it as fast and as hard as you can. This gives the doctor what is called a **Forced Vital Capacity** (FVC) or how much air you are able to blow out at one time. Examination of your test results can show not only how much air you're able to blow, but the speed in which you blow it out. In other words, your lungs may hold 4 liters of air and you blew out 70% of that in the first second. That tells your doctor something about the strength of your lungs as well as the overall volume. So this basic test really can tell a lot about you.

A **Slow Vital Capacity** (SVC) is often coupled with a Forced Vital Capacity to verify the volume measurements. To do this test, you take a deep breath and blow it out slowly. The volume numbers should be the same in both tests. But, for an asthmatic who's having a problem exhaling, there may be a difference.

A common way to test for asthma is to complete the basic spirometry, then to give a bronchodilator, and then repeat the tests. This is done to first determine a baseline reading of the volume and speed, and then to see if the medication helps.

Methacholine Challenge is another test for asthma. This is also known as a **Bronchial Provocation test**. Spirometry measurements are taken of the FVC and the SVC. That provides a baseline. Then you're asked to inhale methacholine as part of a nebulizer treatment. The spirometry testing is repeated. Almost all asthmatics will have a response to the methacholine and will have some bronchial restriction. In other words, your doctor will be provoking your body to have a controlled asthma attack.

The **Maximal Volume Ventilation** test requires a patient to breathe deep and fast for at least ten seconds. It mimics the way we breathe when we do strenuous exercise. This test is known to cause bronchoconstriction and really shouldn't be done if you're an asthmatic. In rare occasions, it's used in asthmatics to document exercise-induced asthma, but it really isn't necessary as part of the average exam.

Diffusion Capacity is really not as bad as it sounds. It's also called **Transfer Factor Testing**. It uses carbon monoxide to determine how gases cross out of the air and into the lungs, and vice versa. You're really only breathing in a little carbon monoxide. You take in a deep breath, hold it for ten seconds, and blow it out again. The testing machine measures the difference between the air you breathed in, and the air you breathed out. The downside to this test is that, to be 100% accurate, smokers should abstain from smoking cigarettes for at least 24 hours. But most doctors forget to tell you that. Of course, if you have pulmonary disease, you shouldn't be smoking anyway!

Helium Dilution and **Nitrogen Washout** is another type of lung volume determination. The procedure varies, but, basically, it measures your total lung capacity. The FVC and SVC measure how much you can breathe in and blow out; this test measures what's left after you blow out and before you breathe in again.

Exercise testing is becoming more common. In its most basic form, you exercise while someone else monitors what happens. A common procedure is the Rest/Exercise Pulse Oximetry. This is a simple procedure that involves putting a portable oxygen saturation monitor (pulse oximeter) on your finger and asking you to exercise. The fluctuations of oxygen levels in your blood are recorded and evaluated. This is often a way that home oxygen therapy is justified to insurance companies.

Exercise testing has also reached more advanced levels. In **Metabolic Testing** you're asked to exercise while breathing through a mouthpiece. The oxygen you breathe in, and the CO_2 you breathe out, are analyzed along with other gases. A determination is made of what goes on metabolically as you exercise, and is recorded. It's unlikely that you'll be asked to do this test – unless you have exercise-induced asthma, or if you're involved in an advanced screening program for food allergies.

Lung Compliance Studies are a measure of the elasticity of your lungs. This measurement may be taken if you're on a ventilator, but it's unlikely that you'll be asked to perform the procedure as a diagnostic test.

Had enough tests? Well, if you've read this far, you automatically pass our test on diagnostic tests!

Part 2
Asthma Basics

Asthma basics

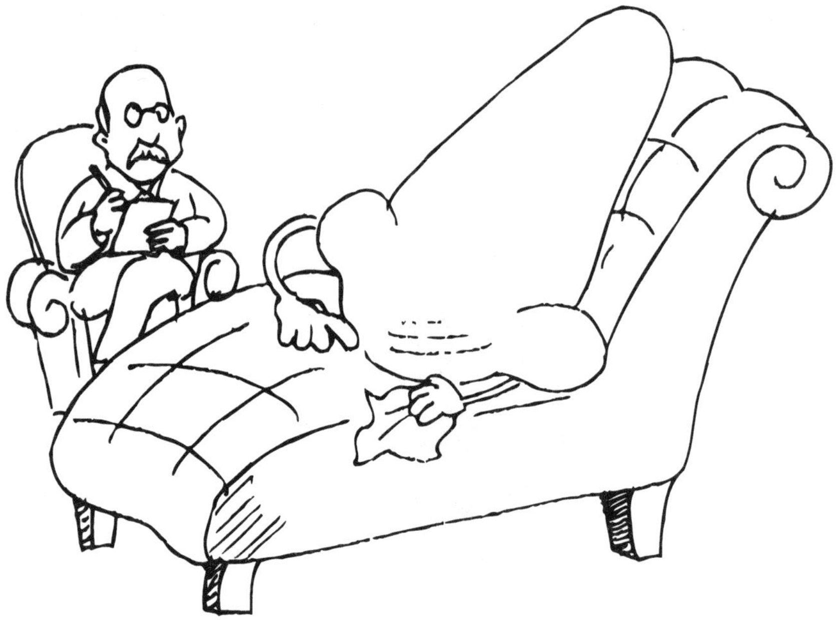

Asthma is a centuries-old problem. It's only been in the last ten to fifteen years, though, that healthcare providers and researchers have learned to effectively deal with the condition.

In the past, asthma sufferers were told that their difficulties breathing were psychological and that they would outgrow it. Many did. Those that didn't were sent to psychiatrists as they got older. Frequently, sedatives were prescribed to help them with their nerves. This may have allayed their fears, but it didn't help their asthma. Today we know that asthma is a chronic inflammatory and restrictive disorder of the airways that can be controlled and effectively managed.

The treatment of asthma has undergone a dramatic evolution in the last decade. As recently as the mid-1980's, many healthcare providers were still treating the occurrence of asthma attacks as isolated episodes. Patients were treated when they had difficulties and were offered little or no preventative therapy.

The focus of treatment has switched, however, with the reclassification of the condition as a chronic process. Many healthcare providers still define asthma as a hyperresponsive airway condition. This isn't wrong, it just isn't telling the whole story. To fully understand the condition, let's look at how an asthma attack happens.

How an Attack Happens

As you breathe, your body takes in air – the good, the bad, and the dirty. The dirty particles are the most troublesome. Researchers still don't know why, but some bodies are more sensitive to particles in the air they breathe than others. To date, heredity is still the strongest predictor as to whether or not an individual is at risk for developing asthma.

While your nose does a good job of filtering out those particles, some of particles do make it to your airway. The airway tissue in an asthmatic is supersensitive to these particles. The particles get into your airway and irritate it. The irritation level can be different for each individual – some people don't ever realize they have asthma. They just report feeling tired and getting short of breath very easily. For others, the irritation causes inflammation. These are the individuals we classically call asthmatics.

Your body typically responds to an irritation by flooding the area with fluid. We are all familiar with the bump that raises when an ant bites us. In the airway, the fluid takes the form of mucus and swelling.

1,2,3 ...

Three things begin to happen in the asthmatic when an irritant enters the airway. First, the airway tube itself begins to fill with fluid and swell like a dry sponge taking up water. This causes the airway to get smaller.

The second process that occurs is the constriction of the muscles in the airway. This may happen as a result of the swelling going on around the muscles or because of the initial irritation. It's still unclear why the airways constrict, but we know that they do. We also know that this is what causes the tight feeling that many asthmatics report. Frequently, patients say that they feel like they are breathing through a straw. This muscular contraction is called bronchoconstriction.

The third process that occurs in the asthmatic airway is an increase in mucus produced by the cells in the airway wall. This is the body's way of flooding the airway and washing out the irritant. Unfortunately, the mucus is often thick and can clog up the airway, making it more difficult to breathe.

Talk The Talk

Medical practitioners love terms. If we can't find one that fits a condition, we make one up. Frequently, there are duplications and overlapping terms used to describe the same illness. An asthmatic airway is also called a hyperresponsive airway, a hypersensitive airway, and a chronic-responsive airway. All that these terms really mean is that there is this underlying inflammatory condition and that the individual's airway is supersensitive.

Muddying the water even more is the onslaught of pharmaceutical companies trying to convince us that their products are unique and special. Then there are the insurance companies that are trying to classify treatments into categories. Don't be alarmed if your healthcare provider uses a different term – just make sure *you* understand what's being talked about. Also make sure your doctor explains your condition and the treatment plan, and that it all makes sense to you.

Triggers

The particles that can irritate an airway are called triggers. A trigger can be smoke, pollution, pollen, dust, mold, animal dander, cockroaches, cold air, warm air, activity, etc. The list is endless. In short, a trigger is defined as anything that precipitates the symptoms of an asthma attack. Different people have different triggers.

Controlling what irritates your airway is the first step in controlling your asthma. By eliminating the trigger, you can greatly reduce the chances of having an attack.

Asthma Severity

Healthcare practitioners love classifying things almost as much as we love new terms. For asthma, there are four levels of severity. But classifying this condition may be a double-edged sword. On the one hand, placing you in a particular category may qualify you for a higher level of reimbursement from your insurance company. That depends on the company. On the other hand, though, it may establish you as a higher risk or as having a preexisting condition. This may affect your future insurability, cause you to pay higher premiums, or cause you to have a waiting period before you're covered by a new insurance plan. In any case, it's unfair to you if your doctor doesn't explain all this to you.

The following categories were developed by the National Heart, Lung and Blood Institute, a division of the National Institutes of Health. They're gaining widespread acceptance and usage. It's important that you, as an asthma sufferer, understand what the categories are.

Mild Intermittent Asthma is the first classification. These patients have experienced symptoms no more than once a week. Their symptoms may last anywhere from a few hours to a few days. They may experience nighttime asthma up to twice a month. In general, these patients feel well and their lung function, when tested, is usually normal. They usually don't require long-term therapy, and use an inhaled relief medication only when symptoms emerge.

Mild Persistent Asthma patients may have difficulty more than once a week, but not every day. Asthma affects their sleep and interrupts their usual activities. These patients may have nighttime asthma two to three times a month. They are usually treated with a long-term preventative medication and use relief medication when symptoms warrant.

Moderate Persistent Asthma patients have daily asthma symptoms. They frequently experience nighttime asthma and their condition interrupts their daily routines. These individuals are usually using long-term preventative medications that may include steroids and taking inhaled medication on a daily basis.

Severe Persistent asthmatics are individuals who have continuous symptoms. These individuals are on very complex treatment regimens. Their physical activity and daily routines are severely inhibited by their condition.

It is important that you understand these categories. You should also note that they are not set in stone. Many different factors can influence your body's response to a trigger. For example, seasonal asthma is not uncommon. Some individuals have difficulty in the fall as mold and pollen counts rise, others in the spring. Knowing that there are different levels of therapy and keeping track of your body's responses will help you and your healthcare provider design your optimum treatment plan.

Taking Control

Prevention is still the best medicine in controlling asthma. In addition to controlling your level of exposure to triggers, you can use a peak flow meter. This is a small device that measures how fast you can blow air out. Measured on a regular basis, you and your healthcare provider can establish a base line range for yourself. When your measurements start to fall below this range, you know there's something irritating and starting to interfere with your breathing.

Your healthcare provider will help you develop a treatment plan based on your peak flow values. For example: when your value falls to a certain range they may encourage you to take a relief medication, at another range you may be asked to come to the emergency room. The goal of peak flow therapy is to assist you in detecting and catching your asthma difficulties before they become severe.

Pharmaceuticals is another area of asthma management that's changing rapidly. In the past we had to rely on the old standbys that relieved the muscular contractions. These drugs were known as bronchodilators.

Today we not only have new types of these medications, but we also have drugs that interrupt the underlying inflammatory process. Medications are also being prescribed in combinations that relieve and even remove the likelihood of an asthma attack altogether. There are new drugs on the market every day. Get to know your pharmacist and ask your doctor questions. Remember, you're still the best judge of what's working – or not working – for you.

As asthma has become very common, there's been an explosion of information and research. The changes are happening so quickly that it's difficult for many healthcare providers to keep up with them all. It's up to you to actively manage and care for your asthma.

Asthma and anxiety

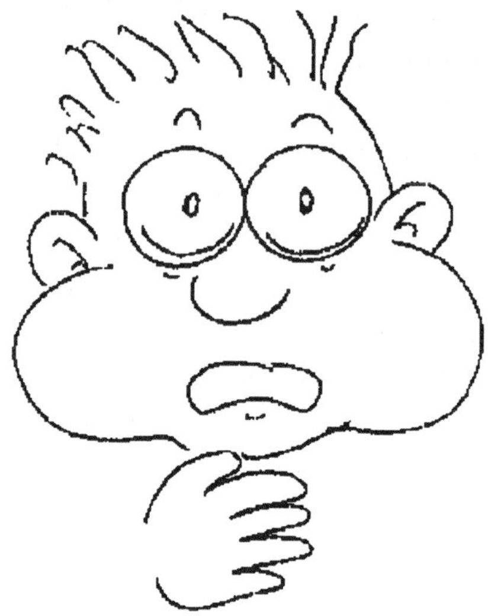

Asthma. We all know it's in your head. Or is it? Historically, the belief has been that it's a psychosomatic illness caused by stress. As early as 1947, psychologists began developing theories that define the asthma-prone personality. Today, researchers are opening new avenues to the origins and causes of the condition. Increasingly, we're learning that there are physiological, as well as genetic, factors involved.

Stress

Anxiety is an inescapable fact of life in the 1990s. As you become anxious, your body responds by pumping more adrenaline into your blood. Your heart begins to beat faster, your breathing rate increases and your senses become keener. This is commonly known as the Fight or Flight Response. It's an alert mechanism built into our bodies to help protect us from dangerous situations. In prehistoric times this mechanism probably saved our ancestors from being eaten by some animal. In modern society, the need to run for your life to avoid becomng lunch is not often experienced.

Our stresses have changed, but our bodies haven't. The Fight or Flight Response is useful in cases of dire emergency. We've all heard stories about superhuman strength. Remember the mother who lifted a car up off her child? Most of us experience mild versions of this response every time we become anxious. And most of us handle the changes that go on in our bodies without difficulty.

For the asthmatic, however, the alteration in breathing patterns caused by the Fight or Flight Response can quickly escalate into a problem. There's also a percentage of people who don't have true asthma, but can develop asthma-like symptoms when placed under certain stresses. These symptoms can escalate into a panic attack if left untreated. And this can be fatal if not handled properly. Most health care providers can't tell the difference between a true asthma attack and a panic attack. All they see is that someone has shown up in the Emergency Room with asthma-like symptoms. The danger is that these patients will be treated as asthmatics, placed on long-term therapy, and spend years taking unnecessary medication. "Anxiety-induced asthma" is a new term that's being used – often interchangeably with "panic attack."

Panic Attacks

A panic attack can come on very suddenly and escalate quickly (usually within 10 minutes). Many patients will report feelings of fear or feeling uncomfortable prior to the attack, but others report no unusual feelings at all. The symptoms of a panic attack can include a pounding, rapid heart rate, sweating, trembling, difficulty breathing, choking or smothering sensations, chest pain, nausea, dizziness, chills or hot flashes; feelings of being detached from your body or seeing yourself from above; and a fear of impending disaster or death.

Any or all of these symptoms can occur as part of a panic attack. Typically, you can be going about your daily routine when your heart begins to beat faster. The other symptoms usually follow quickly. As the outward symptoms progress, changes inside your body occur, as well. Your blood pressure begins to rise. And blood levels of oxygen and carbon dioxide begin to fluctuate as your breathing changes. These two blood levels are important in maintaining balance in your body chemistry, and they play a key role in keeping all of your organs working right.

Your body takes in oxygen when you inhale and uses it as a fuel at the cellular level. It's like the match that adds the spark cells need in order to function. Carbon dioxide is the waste product that's produced when the match is all used up and burns out. It's removed from the body in the air you exhale. When the level of carbon dioxide in the blood goes up, your body breathes faster to get more out and to bring more oxygen in. One of the healthiest examples of this is when you exercise. Your body needs more energy, so it burns more oxygen; the carbon dioxide level goes up, so you breathe faster.

Researchers have begun taking a closer look at how fluctuations in the blood levels of oxygen and carbon dioxide affect asthma and panic attack sufferers. Their goal is to determine the link between the two conditions and develop more effective diagnosis and treatment plans. The present findings outline three basic categories of

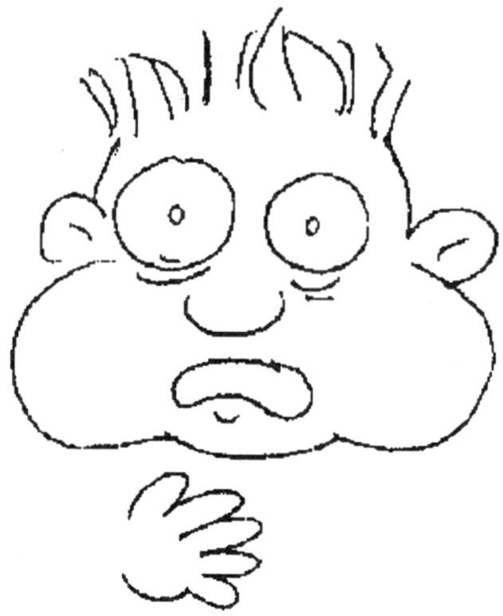

anxiety-induced asthma.

Three Types of Anxiety-Induced Asthma

The first category is **Hyperventilation Syndrome**. This theory isn't new. It was first proposed in 1937. Called HVS, this syndrome compounds itself as it progresses. As you become anxious, you begin to breathe rapidly. The faster you breathe, the shallower your breaths become. You take less oxygen into your blood because there simply isn't enough time to take deep breaths and get the oxygen in. Large volumes of air move in and out of the lungs, but it isn't getting deep enough and it isn't staying there long enough for the oxygen to cross into the blood.

You are, however, flushing the CO_2 or carbon dioxide out of your blood. This causes the blood levels of CO_2 to drop, which is known as hypocapnia. As a result of this drop in carbon dioxide level, the blood vessels throughout your body begin to tighten. This causes a chain reaction of other symptoms. When the blood vessels in your head constrict, you become light-headed or dizzy. In extreme cases, as the CO_2 levels drop, vision becomes affected and you begin to feel as if you're seeing the world through a fog. An impending sense of doom overcomes many people at this point.

You may become even more anxious as the symptoms occur. Your heart beats faster and you even feel as if it's going to jump out of your chest. It's a downward spiral for you if intervention doesn't occur quickly. This condition is usually treated by the classic breathe-in-a-brown-paper-bag method. The bag catches the carbon dioxide that you exhale and allows you to rebreathe it in. This raises the blood levels and begins to break the cycle. This is the syndrome we've all heard described as "all in your head." But studies are now showing that it's not in your head – it's really happening.

Most of us can handle the rapid fluctuation in carbon dioxide levels. However, there's a group of people that cannot. New findings suggest that these people have a blood chemistry that predisposes them to HVS. The normal level of CO_2 in their blood is already lower than average. When they take the first few anxious breaths, their levels drop dangerously and can push them into a full-blown anxiety attack. These studies are not conclusive, but the good news is that deep breathing and training in abdominal breathing can help.

The second category of anxiety-induced asthma also looks at blood chemistry levels. While the first theory dealt with lower blood levels of CO_2, the second theory deals with elevated levels. This theory is also a bit younger. It was first determined in 1967 that *increases* in blood CO_2 levels can also trigger an anxiety attack in some people. This can be stimulated by breathing in higher than normal levels of CO_2. For research purposes, it can also be induced by injecting the patient with lactate. Both result in elevated blood CO_2 levels and a rapid hyperventilation reaction. The subsequent rapid breathing spurs the panic attack.

Researchers don't know why some people are so sensitive to elevated blood levels of CO_2. They do know that when given lactate, or when challenged with a slightly higher mixture of CO_2 in the air they breathe (about 5%), these people develop a choking feeling and have difficulty breathing. Many report that they feel as if they're smothering. Some researchers believe that these people have a low suffocation threshold. When challenged, their bodies send out the false alarm that they're smothering. This triggers the rapid breathing and the panic attack.

These studies are garnering particular interest from researchers in many fields of medicine. Environmentally, we know that our global CO_2 levels are on the rise. From a nutritional perspective, the use of lactate is interesting. Could diet induce asthma and anxiety responses in some people? The only answer we have at the moment is: we don't know. There have been studies in animals that recognize the changes in elevated CO_2 levels. But studies in humans are not complete.

A starting point for researchers is a rare congenital condition called CCHS or **Congenital Central Hypoventilation Syndrome** or Ondine's curse. This is a malfunction of the patient's nervous system which causes a loss of the automatic control of breathing. When someone has this condition the body doesn't respond to the elevated blood CO_2 levels. It doesn't tell the lungs to breathe more and expel the CO_2.

CCHS patients are less likely to have panic attacks, and it's said that they have a high anxiety threshold. This holds true for the small group of CCHS patients who also have asthma. Biofeedback and breath training is encouraged for all people classified with category two anxiety-induced asthma.

The third category of anxiety-induced asthma follows the **Cognitive Behavior Theory**. These are people who experience mild symptoms of difficulty in breathing or rapid heart rate, and it frightens them. In fact, it frightens them so much they become progressively more anxious and scare themselves into having a panic attack. It's a positive feedback cycle, or vicious cycle, that escalates and escalates. The mild symptoms that spur this vicious cycle are called interoceptive cues.

In lay terms, the first two groups of asthmatics have a physiological or body chemistry basis. This last group is, in fact, purely psychological and induced by the people themselves. They feel uncomfortable, it frightens them, and they panic. The third group incorporates the idea that these people have a higher-than-average sensitivity to anxiety. They're very sensitive to abnormal physical feelings and they become anxious.

Diagnosis in this third category can be tricky. Some studies have exposed these patients to elevated CO_2 and lactate levels in a controlled, soothing atmosphere. These patients did not have panic attacks. They also didn't have panic attacks when asked to hyperventilate in a controlled environment. So fluctuations in their blood chemistry didn't induce an attack.

Researchers can't explain what does trigger their symptoms. Another monkey wrench in this group that can't be explained is why these people are occasionally awakened from sleep by panic attacks. All of this makes them prime candidates for behavioral modification therapies, including biofeedback, stress reduction and breath training.

Being unable to breathe is a frightening thing, no matter what the cause. Because symptoms of asthma and anxiety-induced asthma overlap, diagnosis and treatment is complicated. Difficulty breathing causes panic and panic causes difficulty breathing. It's hard to differentiate between the two. Depending on the study you read, anywhere from 6% to 30% of all asthmatics have some type of panic disorder. People with asthma are believed to be more sensitive to the body's sensations and responses. They're encouraged to monitor their own condition.

So, keep track of your peak flows, be aware of how you feel, and speak up when you see your health care provider. Misdiagnosis of a panic attack as an anxiety attack and vice versa can be potentially fatal for an asthma sufferer. If you're an asthma sufferer and know or suspect that you have an anxiety-related condition, tell your doctor! Your physician can help you determine the best treatment and training you require. It's a matter of life and breath. More specifically, it's a matter of *your* life and *your* breath.

LAM: Rare, but NOT asthma

Lymphangiolieomyomatosis. It's a mouthful, isn't it? It's also a rare lung disease that affects women of child-bearing years. The dangerous thing about this disease, known as LAM, is that it's often misdiagnosed as asthma. The women are usually diagnosed with adult or late onset asthma. This mistake results in the patient receiving the wrong treatment, sometimes for years.

There have been 250 known cases of LAM in the U.S. Conservative estimates suggest that there may be as many as three times as many cases undiagnosed, or misdiagnosed as asthma.

The most common complaint is difficulty breathing with exercise or exertion. Occasionally, sufferers will complain of chest pain, and sometimes they will cough up blood. The illness becomes progressively worse over time.

The most painful and life threatening side effect is recurrent pleural effusions and pneumothoraces. That's fluid or air trapped in the chest that doesn't permit the lungs to completely inflate.

We just don't know what causes LAM. It can be diagnosed by open lung biopsy. Basically this means that a physician goes into the person's chest and takes a sample of lung tissue. The sample is examined microscopically. A lung infected by LAM usually reveals infiltration of the pulmonary tissue by smooth muscle tissue cells. The muscle tissue cells are normal in other parts of the body, but, not in the lungs.

The muscle cells then form bundles, and eventually group into cysts. These cysts may show up on a chest X-ray, however a CAT Scan is more likely to assist the physician in presenting a complete picture. When the doctor looks at the CAT scan, the cysts look like blobs or holes. It has an overall Swiss cheese sort of look.

Diagnosis of LAM can also be done by thoroscopy. This procedure requires the physician to look inside the chest with an endoscope. The cysts are usually seen via the endoscope as being evenly dispersed across the lung tissue.

Because LAM affects women of child-bearing years, researchers are searching for a link between the illness and estrogen and other female hormones. None of the women studied to date have had a hormonal abnormality. But, the researchers believe, the correlation between the types of women affected and the illness is too strong to ignore. They are continuing to search for a link. They are also searching to see if there is a genetic link. But there have been no documented cases of a mother and daughter both having LAM.

The other main focus of LAM research is examining the link between the occurence of the pulmonary condition and a benign kidney tumor called Angiomyolypoma or AML. This rare tumor occurs simultaneously in 50% of all LAM cases. Researchers don't know why, but they are looking into it.

Because so little is actually known about the illness, treatment of LAM is not standardized and there are no definitive guidelines for physicians to follow.

Since LAM is usually misdiagnosed as asthma, patients are often started on a course of asthma therapy. As the illness progresses they are less and less responsive to the asthma drugs. Both patient and physician become frustrated, as the drugs don't help and they don't know where to turn. The patients are given stronger and stronger asthma drugs, none of which seem to work.

When the condition is finally diagnosed as LAM, the treatment regimen shifts dramatically. Efforts become more focused on the reduction of estrogen, in an attempt to slow the progress of the muscle fiber growth. This can be done by one of two approaches. The woman's ovaries can be removed. She will likely be placed on some type of low dose hormone replacement therapy and calcium supplements, now that she's at greater risk for developing osteoporosis and other illnesses. Balancing the amount of hormones her body needs and how much is too much to keep the LAM in check can be tricky business.

The other approach to treating LAM is to leave the ovaries intact and to use medication to supplement progesterone levels. This allows a woman's body to naturally suppress estrogen. Each course of therapy has its proponents.

If the LAM progresses to the point that the lungs are non-functioning, a lung transplant is considered. This is a dangerous procedure and, unfortunately, the transplant doesn't cure the LAM. There have been cases in which the LAM develops in the new lung. This suggests to researchers that the origin of the illness lies outside of the pulmonary system. But they don't know where the LAM comes from and they don't understand what motivates the illness to attack the lungs.

LAM patients aren't alone in their battle. The LAM Foundation is located in Cincinnati, Ohio and can be reached at (513) 777-6889. The LAM Foundation works to spread the word and educate physicians, as well as the general public. Besides fighting to find a cure, they have to fight to get people to listen. They offer literature, support and assistance to patients and caregivers.

LAM studies are being funded by the National Heart, Lung, and Blood Institute. They are still in the preliminary stages. No reportable data has been collected yet.

The chance that you were misdiagnosed with asthma when you really have LAM is slim to none. It's a rare condition. But the truth is, we just don't know enough about this illness. Researchers believe it's more common than we think, yet most doctors don't know what to look for.

Asthma and arthritis

Did you ever think your allergies and asthma could be caused by arthritis? Strange as it sounds, it may be true. Scientists are researching a phenomenon called neurogenic switching that may explain links between these conditions. Put simply, neurogenic switching means that irritation at one point in the body may cause an inflammatory reaction at another, unrelated point. In other words, if you stub your toe, your hand may swell up. The body responds to irritation with inflammation.

Inflammation

There are basically two types of inflammation. The first type is called neurogenic inflammation. This occurs when chemicals called neuropeptides are released from a local site in the body, like your toe. These chemicals sound the alarm that an injury has occurred and the body answers with inflammation.

The second type of inflammation is called immunogenic. This is said to occur when an antigen binds with an antibody – like a key fitting into a lock. This is the response that often occurs when an outside irritant, such as an allergen, invades the body. The body's immune system sends in the cavalry to help fight that allergy attack, and inflammation occurs.

Crossed Wires

When neurogenic switching happens, the two types of inflammation get their wires crossed. The body receives the message that an injury has occurred on one line, but instead of the response being sent back along the same pathway, it gets lost and is sent to an unaffected site in the body. The inflammation occurs at this other part of the body.

Scientists are also beginning to believe that this is how anaphylactic reactions occur – for example, when your throat swells and you can't breathe if you're stung by a bee. The theory of neurogenic switching is gaining widespread acceptance and causing researchers to rethink how they treat inflammation. Increasingly, researchers are looking at tried and true arthritis formulas and applying them to asthmatics.

Medications

Gold salt therapy has long been a mainstay of rheumatoid arthritis treatment. The exact mechanism of its action is obscure, but one study showed that it helps asthmatics. In 1978, Muranka, et al, used gold salt therapy with 79 asthmatics for over 30 weeks. 71% of the patients receiving the gold salt showed a marked improvement in their asthma symptoms. In follow-up studies, researchers were able to document a "complete remission" of asthma, and a decrease in the patients' need for glucocorticosteroids.

For some reason, it seems that this work was forgotten for almost 18 years. But today there is a resurgence in gold salt research. Perhaps it was felt that the side effects of gold salt were too uncomfortable. These effects include diarrhea, rashes, and oral ulcers.

Methotrexate (MTX) is another arthritis drug getting a second look. Pharmacologists call this drug an immunomodulator. It regulates the body's inflammatory response. Asthma patients are started on the same regimen as arthritis patients. Studies suggest that MTX has a stabilizing effect on asthma when the drug is taken at low doses. Patients that are seemingly dependent on steroids are able to reduce their dosage of the steroid and possibly stop their use completely when taking MTX.

But like gold salts, there's a problem with side effects. Vomiting, nausea and diarrhea have been noted at the higher dosage. All patients must be monitored for hepatic fibrosis (a liver condition) and neutropenia (a drop in the circulating white blood cell count), regardless of dosage received. The American College of Rheumatology is very concerned about the effect MTX has on a patient's liver. They recommend that lab work be done every 4 to 8 weeks and that patients be closely watched for pulmonary toxicity.

People taking MTX seem to be at risk for interstitial fibrosis and acute pneumonitis. Both can be fatal if left undetected. We do know that an oral folate (a salt of folic acid, a B vitamin) seems to decrease the risk of toxicity, but the studies of side effects are all related to the drug's usage in the treatment in arthritis. Long-term studies on its safety for asthma patients are only now beginning.

Other arthritis drugs being investigated for use in asthma therapy include: **Cyclosporin A**, another immunomodulator; FK506 and Rapamycin, leukotreine inhibitors; and Dapsone. Dapsone is known to decrease the immune system's response to allergens. A very limited study involving ten asthmatics has shown that after 13 months, seven were able to stop their steroid use entirely. Two others were able to decrease their steroid dose by 74%, and one patient didn't respond to the therapy. These are promising results, but obviously, more work needs to be done.

Inflammation is unquestionably a part of life for asthma and allergy sufferers. Re-examining and rethinking old remedies may help us better understand and treat our illnesses. Who says you can't teach an old dog new tricks?

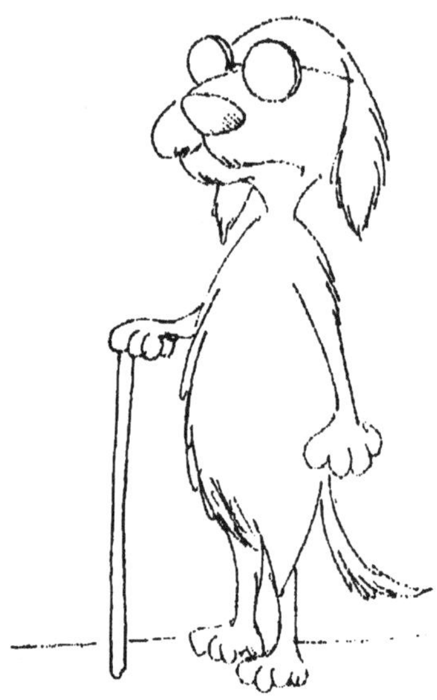

Asthma, allergies, and pregnancy

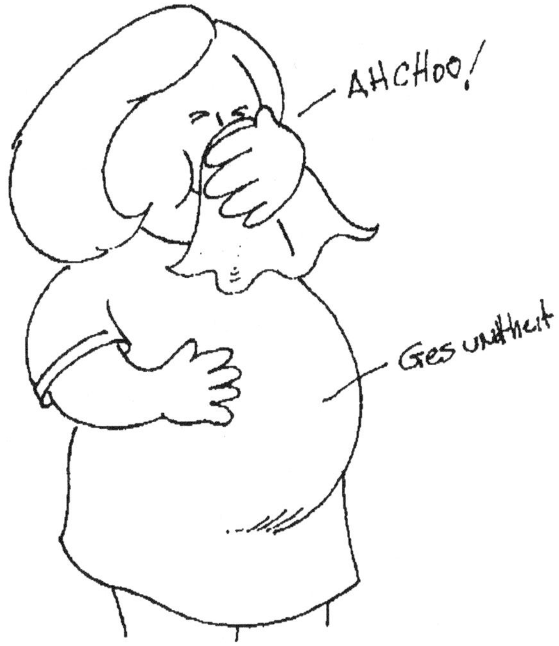

So you're having a baby. Congratulations! But, what about your asthma? Can your allergies get worse because you're pregnant? And what about all that medication you take? These are just some of the questions expectant moms wonder about. Now that you're breathing for two, let's look at what medicine knows.

Allergies and Asthma

About 30% of all pregnant women experience rhinitis and purulent sinusitis during pregnancy. These allergy-like symptoms usually subside after giving birth. Researchers are unsure as to what exactly causes this condition. One theory is that the congestion is caused by the effect of increased estrogen levels circulating in the mother's blood.

Another commonly-held idea is the increased blood volume theory. The woman's body increases the amount of circulating blood in her system to provide nutrients and oxygen for her baby. As this occurs, the smaller vessels in the mother's nose swell. This results in a stuffy, runny, nose. Many women also experience clogged Eustachian tubes ("blocked ears") and occasional dizziness. They report the feeling as being similar to having a cold. For women already suffering from allergies, these added symptoms can make life miserable.

Asthma as a result of pregnancy is rare. But if you already have asthma, chances are your physician won't alter your treatment plan. The most important tool in managing breathing needs during pregnancy is awareness. You're breathing for both you and your baby and it's up to you to monitor your condition. Avoid situations that aggravate or trigger your asthma. Don't smoke. Avoid smoky rooms. If the pollen or spore count is high use the air conditioner, use air filters and stay indoors if possible. If you must venture out, do so in the morning, before the air becomes saturated with car exhaust and pollutants. Avoid people who have colds or the flu. If you haven't had your own flu vaccine, it's recommended that you get it after the first trimester of pregnancy.

The peak flow meter is perhaps the most useful tool we have for managing asthma. Experts recommend keeping a peak flow diary to monitor your condition. Measure your peak flow at least twice a day, and also if you feel any change in your breathing. By doing this, you and your health care provider can establish your baseline.

There's a growing trend toward helping patients develop a step treatment program. This treatment plan utilizes your ideal range and incorporates a graded response to treatment. If your peak flow is within 80% to 100% of your ideal, the regular treatment regimen is continued. If your peak flow falls to 50% to 80% of the ideal, then you begin a predetermined treatment plan. If there's no response, or if the peak flow falls to below 50%, you should take immediate action. This usually includes beta agonist therapy and being seen by a physician.

During Pregnancy

Many expectant mothers report difficulty taking a deep breath. This occurs in both asthmatic and non-asthmatic moms. The exact cause of the feeling is unknown. One theory is that the growing baby pushes up on the mother's diaphragm and prevents her from taking a deep breath. Another idea is that the growing baby's increased demands on the mother's respiratory system require Mom to work harder – and she has difficulty keeping up.

Whatever the cause, most moms get relief when they stop and rest for a few minutes until the feeling passes. Asthmatic mothers must remember not to panic when the feeling occurs. The increased anxiety and emotional upset could escalate into an asthma attack. Check your peak flow and respond in accordance with your step program.

When Baby Comes

About 90% of asthmatic mothers do just fine in delivery. Because there's a 10% chance of an asthma attack during labor, you should continue your medication as usual. It's also important that the nurses and staff taking care of you know that you're an asthmatic. Some drugs commonly given during labor (like morphine) can stimulate a histamine response and aggravate your asthma. There are other drugs available that can be used if the staff is aware of your condition.

Your body is going to go through many changes as you give birth to your baby. Your oxygen needs will double and sometimes triple as you work, not only to breathe for the baby, but also to move him along the birth canal. The added stress and rapid breathing may aggravate some asthmatics. For this reason, oxygen is sometimes given usually via a nasal cannula, which is a small tube that's placed under your nose. If your doctor prescribes this treatment don't be alarmed. It's just a precaution. It only means they're not taking any chances and are taking every possible step to insure all goes well for you and your baby.

A Bundle of Joy

After your baby arrives, if you have asthma you should continue your medication and your peak flow diary. Your body still has many stresses ahead. Your hormone levels will still be fluctuating as your body attempts to return to normal. If you decide to breast feed, your body must also adapt to that. Your physician can help you identify the ideal medication program for breast feeding. There are some medications that are approved for lactating mothers and some that are not. Be sure to doublecheck any drug by asking your doctor, your pharmacist and by reading on your own.

Can asthma and allergy sufferers have normal, healthy babies? Of course! But it's up to you to be an advocate for both you and your baby. Remember – you really are breathing for two.

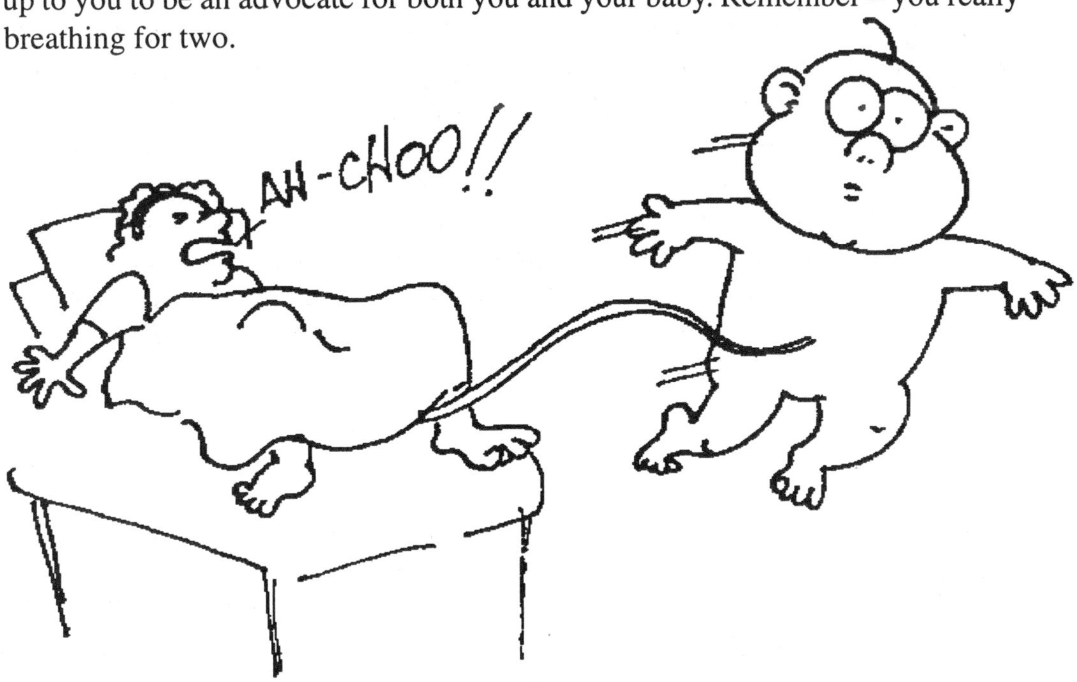

Tips for children with asthma

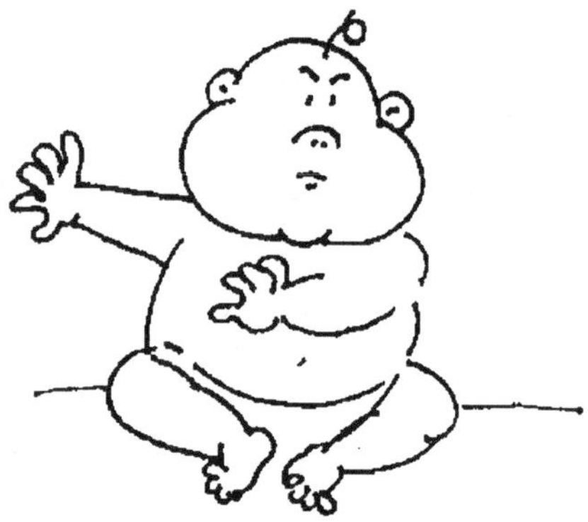

As parents, we worry about our children, even when they're fine. That's part of being a parent. Learning that your child has asthma, or any other type of breathing disorder, makes it worse. How are you going to help your child cope? And how are you going to convince your child to take the treatment?

How your child reacts to nebulizer therapy is going to depend largely on your attitude and how you present yourself. It's frightening when your baby can't breathe. But if you're upset and nervous, he'll pick that up from you.

Make It A Game

Try to make the nebulizer a game: play with it, blow the "smoke" around, laugh. Make it a daily ritual if necessary. Before bedtime, rock the baby and give him the nebulizer. Even on the evenings your child doesn't need the nebulizer, rock him and play with the device. Then when he does need it, he won't be frightened by it.

Many babies don't like to use a mask. They try to pull it off as soon as they are able. So try holding the mask in front of the baby's face without putting the strap around his head. That's less frightening. As your child gets older and becomes more autonomous, use an old nebulizer as a toy so he can give his Teddy bear a treatment.

Use A Timer

What if your sweet baby boy has hit the Terrible Twos? At this age, children have a very short attention span. When asthma makes them feel bad, it gets shorter. Use a timer to help your child "see" his treatment. If he still won't take a treatment, try breaking it into achievable segments. Ask him to take five big breaths and then five more, and still five more until the treatment is completed. Make sure that you give him constant positive reinforcement for his efforts.

MDIs

Some toddlers do well with metered dose inhalers (MDIs), some don't. It all depends on the child. Many physicians ask children to monitor their own peak flows. Believe it or not, teaching a child to do a peak flow measurement is not impossible. It is, in fact, similar to teaching him how to use an MDI. Begin with a party favor or a balloon. Teach him how to blow out on request and show him how to blow in. Only allow him to "play" with the party favor when an adult is around. This will reinforce and emphasize that what he's doing is important and should only be done with supervision. At that age, children are still too young to go it alone. When they're older, they'll understand the difference.

As the child matures and prepares to start school, switching him to an MDI is usually recommended. Begin by teaching him to blow in and out as mentioned above. Continue the nebulizer for the first treatment in the morning and the last treatment in the evening. Use the MDI during the day until he's mastered the technique, providing his asthma is controlled.

Never send him to school with an MDI unless you have first discussed the need and use of the device with his teachers, and the school nurse or principal. While your child may understand its function and use, others won't. The potential that it could be lost or misplaced is too great. The worst thing that could happen is that he'll need it and it won't be handy. Teachers should be kept updated on his condition and any possible situations that could trigger an asthma attack. As he matures, he'll learn what aggravates his condition and, with help from both you and his teachers, he'll learn how to avoid and/or deal with those situations.

Summer Camp

Most state respiratory societies have an annual Asthma Camp in the summer. This is a wonderful opportunity for your child to meet others with asthma and to learn more about his condition. It's also a good opportunity for him to explore new activities (swimming, horseback riding, etc.) with trained professionals nearby. Adolescents also benefit from these programs by learning to be more independent from Mom and Dad, in a safe environment. Breaking away and rebelling a bit is normal for teenagers. At camp, they can learn to be responsible for their own treatment and receive positive reinforcement from peers with asthma.

Learning that your child has asthma is difficult. Helping your child learn to deal with it is even tougher. But it is possible and help is available. There are many groups, including the American Lung Association and Mothers of Asthmatics, that are ready and willing to help. Many hospitals have programs and support groups. You and your child don't have to go it alone.

Exercise-induced asthma

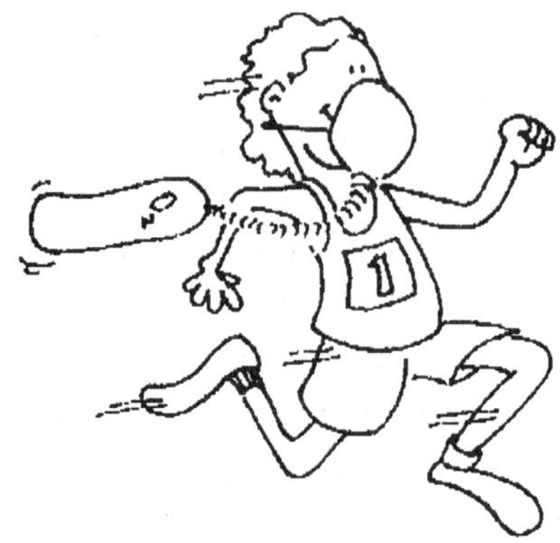

America was thrilled to watch her Olympic athletes go for the gold. But did you know that 10% of our athletes suffer from exercise-induced asthma? Sadly, most health care professionals fail to recognize the signs and symptoms of exercise-induced asthma. And many can't understand that it's different from other forms of asthma. Understanding EIA is just as difficult for sufferers. There are many theories, but no one really knows the cause.

The most widely held belief is that vigorous exercise creates stress on the airway and concurrently increases the metabolic workload that must be supported. The airway becomes overwhelmed and responds by constricting. It's a vicious cycle of aggravation, irritation and constriction.

The Asthmatic Response

The asthmatic response, in essence, feeds and stimulates itself. Most EIA sufferers don't wheeze. They do, however, experience a tightness in their chest. Many report feeling winded or dizzy, and some have abdominal cramps. Symptoms usually appear within 10 to 15 minutes of beginning vigorous activity. They may continue for 30 to 40 minutes after exercise has stopped.

Exercise both aggravates and alleviates the condition. Patients in good physical condition, who exercise regularly, report fewer attacks. Yet exercise also triggers the episodes. Usually you're the best judge as to when and how you should exercise.

Swimming is the most frequently recommended form of exercise for EIA sufferers. Low intensity exercise – such as walking or isometric exercises – is usually also a good choice.

While many still enjoy running (a good aerobic choice), it does seem to aggravate the condition. But if running is your goal, it's not impossible. Specialists in sports medicine can work with you and your physician to develop a step-by-step training program. These training programs usually begin with walking to help improve your overall physical fitness and stamina. As your overall condition improves, you may progress to jogging and then to running.

Many EIA sufferers enjoy prolonged endurance-type exercises with little ill effect. These activities, like downhill skiing, create a constant yet stable elevated stress level on the body.

Perhaps the worst form of exercise for those with EIA is the kind that usually requires high intensity, rapid bursts of activity like basketball or baseball. But these sports aren't impossible, either. If you really enjoy shooting hoops, your health care provider can help you develop a conditioning program that will enable you to do so.

The key to success, however, is sticking to that program. As non-EIA sufferers know, that usually isn't a lot of fun. It's particularly hard on children. It's important that they understand that they must cope with their condition on a daily basis. On one day they may be able to play 15 to 20 minutes, nonstop. On other days they may not be able to do so.

The Secret To Success

Is there a secret weapon to dealing with EIA? Yes. Breathing! Learning breath control and proper breathing techniques is crucial, say experts. Olympic athletes with EIA, like swimmer and gold medalist Tom Dolan, learn quickly that slow deep inhalations through the nose warms and humidifies the air.

This reduces stress and shock on the body and reduces the chance of an asthma attack. On cold or dry days, exercise indoors if possible. If it's not possible, try wearing a scarf or mask to hold the warm moist air in. If exercising outdoors is the only alternative, then do so in the early morning hours before the air becomes congested with car emissions and pollutants. Air pollution and allergens like pollen are known to aggravate the condition.

It's not unusual for athletes with EIA to take more time warming up and cooling down. This gives their body a better opportunity to adapt to the metabolic demand and the changing environment. Staying hydrated and eating a balanced diet helps many. But eating before exercising can also trigger a response. EIA patients are encouraged to abstain from bananas, nuts, shellfish, eggs, and milk products for at least two hours before exercising. Taking care of yourself and listening to your body are the best warm-ups for exercise with EIA.

Our Olympic athletes collected their medals despite suffering from the same aggravating illnesses we do. Asthma doesn't slow them down, and it doesn't have to slow you. Follow their lead, and you can be a champion, too, in whatever you do.

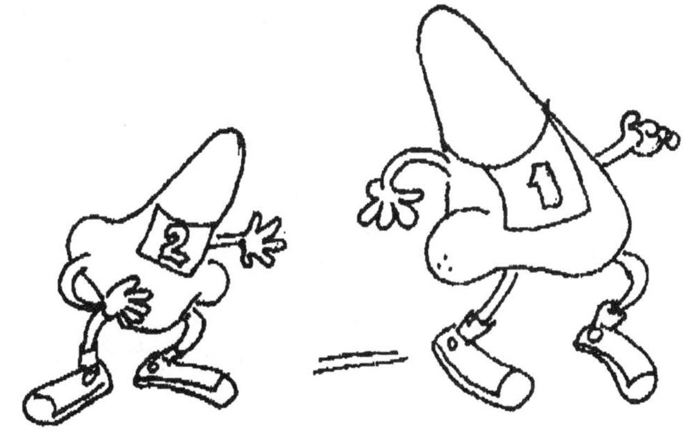

Is it asthma, or Vocal Cord Dysfunction ?

What is the single thing that we do every day that both defines and limits us? It's the one thing most of us don't give a second thought to, and yet it has a profound impact on our careers, our social lives and the types of individuals who are a part of our lives.

The answer is easy. It is speaking. Most of us don't think for a moment about our speaking voice and yet, as soon as we open our mouths, people evaluate and make judgment calls about our capabilities, our education and our socio-economic status.

We also rarely give a thought to our voice box. But misfunctioning of the voice box can result in more than a little hoarseness or a sore throat. Studies are showing that Vocal Cord Dysfunction (VCD) is an undiagnosed problem for many Americans.

Vocal Cord Dysfunction mimics the signs and symptoms of asthma in many patients. Proper diagnosis is a difficult and tricky procedure. Many physicians don't even consider that a component of VCD may be present, and patients are misdiagnosed as difficult-to-control asthmatics. They may endure extensive and heavy drug regimens for years without a definitive diagnosis. The National Jewish Center for Immunology and Respiratory Medicine reports that 30% of their adult patients referred for refractory asthma have both VCD and asthma. Amazingly, 10% have VCD exclusively.

The Larynx

To fully understand VCD, let's take a quick look at how the larynx works. The larynx, or voicebox, is more than just a box that air passes through on its way into and out of the lungs. It's located at the back of the throat, and has three jobs. The first is to protect the trachea or windpipe. A cartilage-like flap called the epiglottis does this. This flap closes over the larynx and seals off the windpipe when you swallow – to prevent food from getting into your airway. The epiglottis also plays a key role in the second part of the larynx's duties. It keeps air in your lungs. When you hold a deep breath, it's the larynx that contracts and keeps the air in your lungs. The third function of your larynx is phonation, or speaking.

Let's take a quick tour of the larynx and see how it lets you speak. Inside, there are two sets or folds of tissue. These are the vocal cords. The true vocal cords are pearly white. The false vocal cords, also known as the vesicular folds, are attached more sideways and assist the true cords in manipulating the airway. In older textbooks these are sometimes referred to as the superior cords (the true cords) and the inferior cords (the false cords).

A complex series of muscles and cartilage allow us to manipulate our vocal cords. The extrinsic or external muscles are divided into two categories. The first set of extrinsic muscles is the infrahyoid group. These four muscles pull the larynx and the hyoid bone down toward the chest. The second set of extrinsic muscles is also composed of four muscles, but these muscles have the more complex job of pulling the larynx up and from front to back in the neck. To feel these muscles in action gently place your hand on your neck and swallow. You will feel your larynx being lifted and pulled toward the back of your neck.

Inside the larynx, cartilage also helps in manipulating the cords. Here's where we get down to the nitty-gritty of speech. Sound is produced by air passing through the cords. Adduction is the process of closing the cords, and abduction is the process of opening them. Air passing through the cords causes them to vibrate, and a sound is produced. The tension of the cords, as well as the amount and speed of air passing through them, and the distance between the two cords (the degree of abduction or adduction), is what causes the variance in sound.

Male vocal cords are usually a little longer and thicker than female vocal cords. This accounts for the difference in the depth of the male voice.

Ideally, during normal breathing, the cords open and flatten out against the walls of the larynx during inspiration. During exhalation, they actually move toward the center of the larynx, but still maintain the glottal space.

VCD

In the case of VCD, the cords do not move in these patterns and an obstruction to airflow is created. The individual seems to wheeze. The sound is almost the same as an asthmatic wheeze. But it's not the result of bronchial constriction that's seen in classic asthma. It's caused by laryngeal contraction or dysfunction. In many instances, you can hear the sound by listening with a stethoscope over the larynx itself. The sounds will be distant over the other airways and lung fields. This is different from asthmatic wheezing, which is usually heard in the airways.

VCD is diagnosed by a procedure called Laryngoscopy. After spraying a mild anesthetic down your throat, the physician takes a scope, looks down your airway, and watches the vocal cords in action. A videotape is often made at the same time, and you can see an instant replay of your vocal cords working. (To definitively diagnose the problem, the procedure should be performed during a wheezing episode.)

A Pulmonary Function Study may also be performed. This test will incorporate methacholine bronchial provocation. The practitioner will ask you to breathe in a gas called methacholine, then he/she will record your airway's response. This is the definitive way to diagnose any asthmatic condition and may assist in determining if there is an asthmatic component to your condition. It will not definitively diagnose the VCD. Only laryngoscopy will do that.

Treatment

The treatment of VCD is just as tricky as the diagnosis. There are many different causes and types of the disorder. More important than delineating all the intricate details, is understanding that a thorough history can help you and your doctor define when the episodes occur and what triggers them.

If you think VCD is a component of your asthma, begin to keep a diary of when your attacks occur, where you are at the time, and what you're doing. Your healthcare provider will need this information.

A very interesting parallel has arisen between panic attacks and VCD. However, there haven't yet been studies performed to determine if there's a link between the two disorders. Most VCD researchers do recognize that there's a psychological component to their patients' conditions. Many have recommended psychotherapy, relaxation therapy, and biofeedback as treatment options for some of their patients. Most recommend speech therapy for proper retraining of the laryngeal muscles. If you think there may be a connection in your case, again, begin to keep a diary and discuss it with your physician.

VCD seems to occur most often in women between the ages of 20 and 40. They report feelings of wheezing and tightness of the throat (not chest) and may exhibit psychological tendencies toward depression, anxiety, and perfectionism (sounds like that panic attack profile doesn't it?). VCD has been reported in children, but hasn't been definitively studied. Clearly, we need more research into this disorder. If the numbers from The National Jewish Center for Immunology and Respiratory Medicine are indicative of a cross section of our asthmatic population, the number of misdiagnosed asthmatics may be significant. Proper diagnosis could spare you from years of unnecessary, intensive asthma regimens that don't really treat what's wrong.

Part 3
Allergy Basics

The basics of allergies

What are allergies? Boiled down to basics, allergies are the over-reaction of your body's immune system to a substance that's considered foreign to your body. Your body becomes extremely sensitive – to something which most people aren't sensitive to at all.

Of course, it's a much more complicated process than you (or scientists) could ever have imagined.

Phase 1

Allergies operate in several stages. The first stage is called sensitization. Your body becomes sensitized to an allergen (the thing you're allergic to, such as ragweed) when it enters your body and becomes an antigen – a protein the body identifies as foreign.

The antigen kicks off the immune response. T-cells are alerted and rush to the scene. They call for help from the B-cells, which stimulate plasma cells to produce IgE antibodies specifically designed to fight that antigen. Your body is now sensitized, meaning it will be ready to fight off that particular antigen the next time it shows up. The antibodies will be ready to go to work, and the body will have a "roadmap" for quickly producing more. The IgE antibodies tie or attach themselves to mast cells, which also carry histamine.

Phase 2

Phase 2 is what we call the clinical disease phase. It's divided into two stages: early and late inflammation. When the allergen shows up again (say, next year's ragweed season), the mast cells explode, releasing antibodies and histamine. Histamine travels through the blood vessels to the nerves and glands, triggering the whole inflammatory process. Histamine is what causes the notorious allergic symptoms of sneezing, itching, congestion, and watery eyes. It opens the blood vessels and causes swelling and bronchial spasms. Antihistamines stop the reaction by blocking the histamine receptor sites, the places where histamine hooks up to do its dirty work.

Every time you come in contact with that allergen, your body will produce more antibodies, and have more mast cells ready to explode. That means more histamine surging through your system.

If this cycle continues, a late-phase reaction occurs, with more little guys known as eosinophils, basophils, monocytes and lymphocytes being produced. At this point, you'll almost certainly show a positive skin test for the allergen.

During the late-phase reaction, your body is so primed waiting for the allergen that it explodes in a frenzy of hyperresponsiveness. More histamine is released than ever and you suffer like never before.

Sometimes late-phase inflammation clears up on its own. That's called resolution. More often, though, it leads to a chronic allergy problem that's considered irreversible. It can also lead to complications.

Two Types of Reactions

Let's go a little bit deeper. There are two types of allergic reactions. Antibody-mediated reactions are the ones we just described, which involve antibodies circulating through your system. They usually occur within minutes of contact with the allergen, and usually disappear within an hour. This type of reaction includes anaphylactic shock, which is an extremely severe – in fact, life-threatening – form of allergy. Anaphylaxis builds over time. The more you're exposed to the antigen, the greater the reaction will be. The sensitivity increases with repeated exposure.

Antibody-mediated reactions can include allergies to bee stings, food allergies to strawberries, chocolate and shellfish, pollen allergies, asthmatic reactions, and some drug allergies, including allergies to antibiotics such as penicillin.

The other kind of allergic response is called cell-mediated. They start several hours after contact with the allergen, and may last for several days. The reaction usually consists of skin inflammation or a rash. Allergens which cause cell-mediated responses include fungus, parasites, chemicals, and poison ivy.

Cell-mediated responses have to do with the T-lymphocyte cells. Symptoms include skin inflammation such as little red bumps, swelling, and itching. Cell-mediated allergies may be induced by contact with nickel, formaldehyde (found in some new rugs and insulation), drugs, cosmetics, chlorogenic acid (in fruits, vegetables and coffee beans), and the chemical substance in poison ivy and poison oak.

Since allergies usually involve a sensitivity to a protein, food proteins are frequent causes of allergies. Elimination of those proteins from the diet is the quickest way to control food allergies. A food allergy may not be the problem, though. Where an allergy will result in a full-blown *immunological* response when even a small amount of the food is eaten, a food sensitivity involves an abnormal *physiological* response. In this case, you'll only have an adverse reaction if you eat more of the offending ingredient than your body will tolerate.

Other common allergens include proteins in springtime tree pollens, summertime grass pollens, fall ragweed and leaf mold, dust mite feces, cockroach allergen, cat saliva, dog dander, human dander, latex, and many types of molds.

What is it you're allergic to? Pinpointing the cause is always a challenge, but an allergist can run tests to find the worst offenders.

Immunotherapy – Allergy Shots To You ...

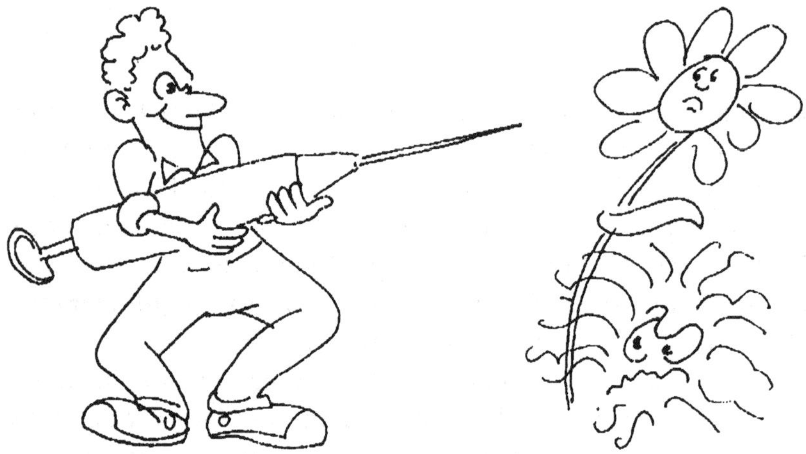

Immunotherapy. The word itself sounds like something out of a bad science fiction novel. The older term for this treatment is even worse: Desensitization. Most of us call it allergy shots. For millions of sufferers, the shots are a godsend. The treatment itself is not difficult to understand, but even after seventy-five years it's still controversial.

If we accept the idea that allergies are caused by exposure to an allergen or irritant, immunotherapy makes sense. Basically, it's the practice of injecting someone with a small amount of allergen over a long period of time. The body gets used to having the allergen around, it learns to live with the allergen, and a tolerance develops. Once this tolerance level is established, the patient may be periodically given a booster shot to maintain immunity. This is known as the maintenance dose or level. The therapy can be effective for both asthma and allergy sufferers. The most common aeroallergens (airborne allergens) for which people in the U.S. receive immunotherapy are house dust mites, mold spores, and pollen from trees, grasses, and weeds.

The treatment includes injecting an extract of the allergen itself. This is the first criticism many have of the practice. The strength and potency of the allergen extract is not standardized in all cases. In other words, one bottle of extract may be twice or even three times as strong as another, even though the labels are the same. (The federal government has begun a program to standardize extracts. Grass allergen extracts, for example, have now been standardized.)

Allergen extract products can vary in strength from lot number to lot number of the same product. This has caused complications. Patients have had severe allergic reactions to improperly given or imprecisely-dosed allergen extract injections.

There are also reports of people receiving lethal doses of allergen extract. The skill (or lack of skill) of the practitioner obviously plays a part. Physicians not well-versed in immunotherapy have given injections that caused serious complications.

Allergy Shots

Allergy shots should only be given by licensed allergists or immunologists. These are the physicians that have the highest, most up-to-date training in the practice. It's interesting to note that in the United Kingdom, the practice of immunotherapy has been banned completely. They've had 26 deaths since 1957 that were directly related to immunotherapy. Many of those who died were given the injections by general practitioners who had neither the equipment nor the skills to manage the severe allergic reactions that followed.

In the U.S., we've had 32 deaths related to immunotherapy injections between the years 1945 and 1985. In the UK, critics point to the unnecessary deaths at the hands of unskilled practitioners and have enacted legislation. We have not done so in the U.S.

You are strongly advised to question your health care providers and demand that they be skilled as well as qualified, and that their training be up-to-date. That's how serious this issue has become.

If you're considering immunotherapy, you should undergo skin testing and screening before initiation of the regimen. A tentative dose schedule should be thoroughly discussed with your doctor. If you're allergic to more than one allergen, the allergen extracts can usually be mixed into one injection without complications.

Immunotherapy

There are three recognized regimens of immunotherapy: The first is Co-seasonal, and it's the least effective of the three. This is a course of treatment that's begun *as* you are experiencing allergic symptoms. The problem is that by the time you start your shots, you've already been exposed to a high level of the allergic antigen – so much that it's brought you to the doctor. Exposing your body to more of the allergen in the form of an injection doesn't make you feel better. And it doesn't alleviate your problems.

Preseasonal therapy is the second regimen. This is a series of injections that's begun three to six months *before* you start to experience symptoms. In other words, if you know you're allergic to spring grass pollens, then you'd begin your shots in November or December. It's kind of like gearing up for the bad season. Shots are usually given weekly, until you reach your tolerance level. The shots are stopped after the season and then repeated again the next year. This regimen is effective, and used by some doctors. The current thinking from the "experts" is that while this works, it's not ideal.

The ideal form of immunotherapy is **Perennial** or year- round. It's now believed that patients who show improvement through three consecutive years of perennial therapy are able to stop the injections and yet still have the immunologic relief of symptoms.

When Should You Get Your Shots?

Okay, so you and your health care provider have discussed the regimen that's right for you. The next topic of discussion is the frequency of the individual shots. The most common frequency or Standard therapy, as it's called, is weekly. You're started on a low dose of allergen extract in the initial injections. Over time, the dosage is gradually increased – as is the time interval of the shots – until a maintenance dose is established. The shots are then often spaced out to bi-weekly, then monthly, etc. It usually takes three to five months to achieve a maintenance level. (An alternative schedule might be suggested by your doctor, though.)

Your doctor may suggest a **Rush Immunotherapy** schedule. This calls for more frequent shots; at least bi-weekly. A One-Month Rush (Cluster) schedule is another alternative: You'll visit the physician once or twice a week, but receive two or three injections per visit. The additional injections are usually given between 30 minutes and two hours later. You'll hit the maintenance level in as little as two to four weeks with this plan, which is useful for those who have a busy schedule or live a great distance from their doctor. The benefit of both the Rush and the Cluster Schedules is that it allows your maintenance dose to be achieved faster than the standard weekly schedule.

There are even more rapid plans. With **6-Day Rush Immunotherapy**, you're admitted to a hospital and given eight shots a day for six days. If there is a reaction, you'll get treatment and then continue on the schedule. With the 1-1/2 Day Rush, you get eight injections over 1-1/2 days, on an outpatient basis. Maintenance is achieved at the end of the second day. And when these Rush plans aren't rushed enough, there's the 1-Day plan: 8 injections over 6 hours. Where snakebite venom is involved, a 1-1/2 *Hour* rush is used, with 12 injections over 90 minutes.

Rush programs are more commonly used in Europe. American allergists are just beginning to explore the possibilities. While the Rush plans may turn out to be cheaper and more convenient for you, between 14% and 30% of patients have a systemic reaction, usually more than 30 minutes after the last injection (and particularly in asthmatics). These reactions may include hives or a rash, generalized itching, sneezing and increase in typical allergy symptoms. The reaction could also be more severe, including wheezing, shortness of breath or tightness. In the worst reactions, anaphylaxic reactions occur, and even a heart attack. These are usually preceded by a sensation of just not feeling right.

Avoiding Complications

To avoid complications from non-standard dosages of extract, most doctors use a graduated system. First of all, each patient should have his or her own bottle of allergen extract. These bottles should be kept in the refrigerator at your doctor's office. Every time a new bottle is opened, your practitioner should start you with a smaller-than-normal dose. They gradually increase the dose with each injection until you reach your normal dosage again.

Don't be afraid to ask your doctor to explain this. It's your body that's getting injected with this stuff. And it's your life they're playing with.

Here's another thing to think about. If you've been on your maintenance dose for twelve months and are still experiencing allergic symptoms, your case should be re-evaluated. You may also want a second opinion.

Some people experience reactions from the injections. A small red bump at the injection site is normal. More serious reactions include a runny nose, tearing, nasal congestion, bronchospasm or wheezing, an itchy rash or hives, and all the symptoms you'd associate with an allergic reaction. The previously-mentioned more serious complication of death is possible, as is a very severe asthma attack for some sufferers.

If you're already on your maintenance dose of allergen extract and you become pregnant, don't worry. You should discuss your case with both your obstetrician and your immunologist. But many women continue their therapy without complications or ill effects to their baby.

Alternatives

Finally, for those of us who don't like needles, there may soon be alternatives. Oral, sublingual (under the tongue) and topical creams are all being tested. The initial work on oral (pill) therapy has been done on birch bark extract. The effectiveness of this route is now being examined on house dust mite extract. So far, researchers have found that in order to be as effective as injections, immunotherapy by one of these alternative routes requires a significantly higher dose of antigen extract.

The final criticism of traditional immunotherapy is that it's expensive. There's hope that ongoing research will develop more cost-effective alternatives.

Immunotherapy has been around for most of this century. There are patients who swear by it, and others who hate it. In the hands of an experienced, licensed practitioner, it can be effective. It's up to you to make the choice that's best for you, and it's your right to question and refuse immunotherapy if you're not comfortable with your practitioner. The most important second opinion is your own.

References: U.S. Mortality statistics extracted from: Lockey, R.F. et al., Fatalities from Immunotherapy and Skin Testing, J. Allergy and Clinical Immunology 79:660, 1987. UK mortality statistics extracted from: Committee on the Safety of Medicines. Desensitizing Vaccines. Br. Med Journal 293:948, 1986

Dust Mites: More than you want to know

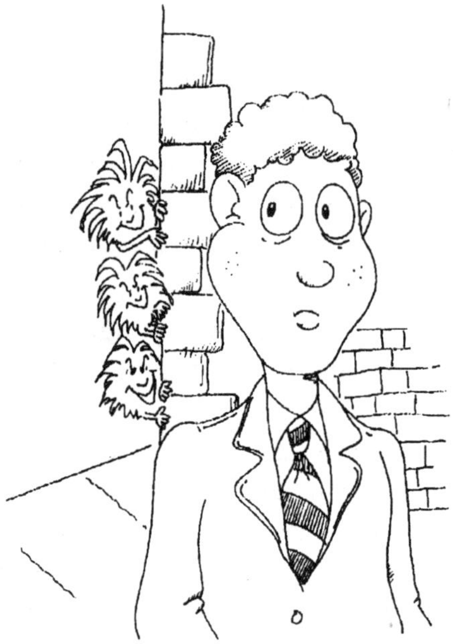

If your allergy or asthma symptoms last all year 'round, you're probably allergic to something in your house. If you live in a major city in the U.S., from Chicago eastward, you could be allergic to the German cockroach, which can result in asthma. If you live in the mountain states (or Scandinavia), and have asthma, you're most likely to be allergic to dog or cat allergen. According to studies, pollen is not usually an independent risk factor for asthma – alone, pollen generally won't trigger an asthmatic episode.

If your allergy problem can't be tied to the outdoor pollen count, and you've eliminated the dog, cat and roach populations as the cause, you're reduced to two choices: you're allergic to human dander (yes, allergic to someone else in the house) ... or you're allergic to dust mites.

While allergy to human dander is possible (although the test for it was withdrawn from the market due to FDA fears of spreading AIDS through the allergy serum) it's much more likely that your problem is due to dust mites.

There are quite a few different species of mites around the world which live in people's houses. A database of global distribution and abundance has been recently established to build a better picture of where and when dust mites affect people.

The Dirt on Dust Mites

Dust mites are arthropods, insects with jointed legs and segmented bodies. In the southern U.S. (plus South and Central America and Asia), the chief offender is *Blomia tropicalis*. Other mites include various *Dermatophagoides* species, *Lepidoglyphus destructor*, and *Euroglyphus maynei*.

They were first identified as a major source of allergens in house dust in 1962.

Mite research continues at a rapid pace, but there's still quite a bit to learn. Thus far, the specific allergens which cause allergies have been identified, and we basically know how they're produced by the mite. These include allergens called Group 1 through Group 10, plus Der p 4, Der p 6, Der p 8, Der p 9, and Eur m 1, Blo t 5, and Lep d 2. The Der refers to *Dermatophagoides* species, the Eur to *Euroglyphus* and Lep to *Lepidoglyphus*. The allergens have been identified and cloned, and a DNA sequence identified. Even the biological function of many of these substances has been identified. Your body can be sensitive to any one of these allergens – or several.

The dust mite lives its life like many other insects. It starts as an egg, hatches into larvae, develops into a nymph, and then grows into an adult, which lays eggs.

Important factors controlling the mite population include outdoor climate, indoor climate, and building characteristics. Humidity and temperature seem to be the most critical factors. Mites live best in warm, humid conditions. They live in a nest, which protects them against short-term variations in humidity. And they hate the light.

House dust mites require greater than 50% relative humidity, and a temperature of more than 70° F. to grow.

Mites eat human skin flakes, which is why mite-allergic people need to encase their mattresses. We're always shedding little pieces of skin, and the mites that live in your mattress will enjoy the meal while you're asleep. An encasement can keep them closeted in the mattress, while keeping your skin scales away from their dinner table.

Mites can also live on fungi in the home, and many other complex food sources, so encasement alone won't solve your problem.

Mite allergen tends to settle out of the air. But the times that it's airborne are when you're most likely to suffer an allergic reaction.

Mite control isn't that difficult; however, it isn't easy for most people to make the effort to transform their homes into a low-mite residence. The ultimate solution is to get rid of your wall-to-wall carpets and upholstered furniture, reduce the humidity in your home, and minimize your bedroom furniture, encasing pillows and mattress. No stuffed toys allowed, either!

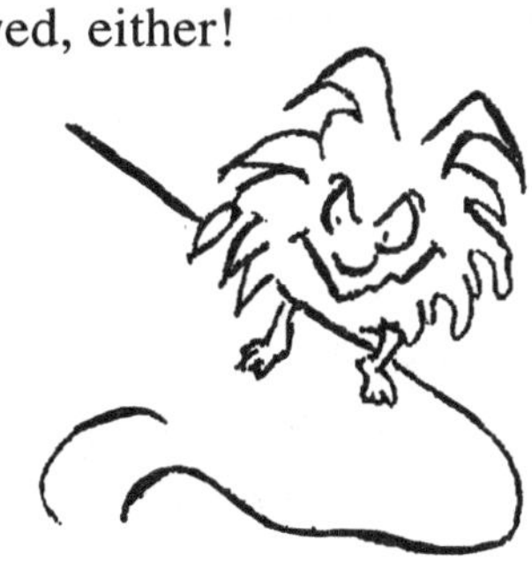

Eliminating Mite Allergen

You can get mite allergen under control. It's not that tough, but it does take a little bit of effort. Let's look at each of the problem areas in your house, and see what you can do to improve your mite control.

Carpets and sofas are primary reservoirs of allergens, humidity and dust mite food. Allergens, from pollen to animal dander to dust mite droppings, are trapped in the carpets, only to rise again as people walk through or vacuum. Moisture is trapped by the fibers of the carpet and the pad, particularly if the carpet is laid over a concrete floor. Because humidity seems to be necessary for mites to thrive and reproduce, carpets are a big problem. In addition, your carpets trap all sorts of food items which mites like. So the carpet is a major breeding ground for dust mites.

This phenomenon is relatively recent. Before the advent of vacuum cleaners, everyone used rugs. Depending on where in the world you lived, these were taken outside and cleaned by beating or laying out in the sun or even in the snow. All of these methods are effective at cleaning the rugs and killing mites.

Today's wall-to-wall carpets lead to the still-unanswered question: Can you kill mites in a carpet which remains on the floor? Some allergy scientists believe that when a carpet is treated, mites will just dig themselves deeper into the carpet or the pad to escape the chemicals. They later resurface when it's safe, and go about their business.

Sofas are another problem area for dust mites. Encasements for just below the fabric area are on the horizon. Recovering with a finely woven polyester fabric blocks cat allergen as well as mite allergen. Treatment with an acaracide or tannic acid remain the main tools.

Vacuuming

Another question is whether vacuuming really does any good. These same skeptics report that all wall-to-wall carpets steadily increase in weight with time. Evidently, vacuum cleaners aren't able to extract all of the material which accumulates in the carpet. This debris in the carpet provides the material mites use for building nests and for feeding. When the mites retreat to their nests, mite-killing acaracides don't touch them.

Steam Cleaning

What about steam cleaning? Again, according to the skeptics, steam cleaning is not designed to reach the bottom layers of the carpet, which are often not colorfast. Water at the bottom tends to bring up colors as well as old stains. (And, there's the question of whether the moisture introduced by the steam cleaner enables mites and molds to breed more quickly.)

Chemicals

There are various products on the market that will kill mites. Among them are abamectin, pirimiphos methyl, benzyl benzoate and tannic acid. Some experiments have shown that benzyl benzoate (Acarosan brand) or pirimiphos methyl will kill mites in a day. But the question remains, just because a substance will kill mites in the laboratory, will it kill them in a residential carpet or sofa?

Most of the acaracides (mite-killers) use benzyl benzoate. It is safe for people, as evidenced by its use as a preservative in food (remember the "less than 1/10 of 1% benzoate of soda" on your grape soda label?). This chemical is available as a moist powder, as a foam, and as a liquid mixed with tannic acid. Tests have indicated that the foam seems to be ineffective on mattresses and sofas.

The powder works better, if it's applied right. The proper technique is to sprinkle the powder on, brush it in, leave it overnight, and brush it in again before vacuuming. A study has shown that it will have a significant effect on dust mite populations for up to 3 months.

Tannic acid is the acid found in tea. It has been used for centuries, and works by denaturing the protein molecules. Since most allergens are proteins, it helps improve conditions by denaturing the allergens.

While tannic acid works well on low concentrations of cat allergen, it was ineffective in a study where it was applied to high concentrations of cat allergen. Further, where cat allergen was present, the tannic acid didn't work as well against the proteins in dust mite allergen. If you have cats, tannic acid can help reduce the total load of allergens, including cat allergen and dust mite allergen.

For best results, first reduce the amount of allergenic proteins in the carpet – by cleaning the carpet – before you apply the tannic acid. Then use a 3% concentration instead of a 1% concentration, if you can. Treat monthly for best results, as the mite levels start to rise again after a week.

Tannic acid has a reputation for staining white carpets, so try it on a hidden spot first. And be extra careful when using it on a basement carpet or on one that's over concrete. The dampness combined with the tannic acid can bring out old stains. And some people report feeling nauseous after using it.

Tannic acid doesn't have a long-term effect, though after it dries out it can be reactivated with moisture, such as that from a steam cleaner. And it has no effect on live mites, just on the mite allergen.

That leads to a distinction which you must understand when thinking about dust mites. Your allergy isn't to the mite itself, but to various proteins and enzymes put out by the mite. Several of these are found in the mite feces. And since the mite often eats its own feces, the proteins are concentrated – and become more potent allergens – each time they pass through the system. So, killing the mites won't eliminate the mite allergen, but it will keep more allergen from being produced. The goal, then, is to kill the mites *and* denature or remove the feces/allergens.

A newer treatment for killing dust mites is the use of borate powders, which are related to borax and boric acid. These powders are applied to the carpet and dry out the environment where the mites live. First used with success for roaches (boric acid) and fleas (polyborate), these powders have now been approved by the EPA for killing mites. (Note that another recent study showed that almost all of the allergen is at the bottom of the carpet – a place that vacuuming, steam cleaning, and most acaracides can't reach. And remember, too, that killing mites will only prevent new allergen from being made – it won't denature existing allergen.)

Dehumidifying

Another recent treatment is a large built-in dehumidifier which automatically keeps your house's relative humidity below the level where dust mites are active. A recent study shows that the Therma-Stor whole house dehumidifier is an extremely effective method for controlling mite populations as well as mold.

Not quite as effective is the use of your central air conditioning to reduce the temperature and humidity. Because air conditioners are not designed with humidity reduction in mind, this is a far less effective method. (Running ventilation fans in bathrooms and the kitchen will help lower the humidity level, too.)

Mattresses, Pillows, and Curtains

Don't forget the encasement for your mattresses and pillows. Wipe down the encasement every two weeks with a damp rag. Wash all bedding, including blankets, pillowcases and mattress pads *every week.* While it was previously accepted that hot water was necessary to kill mites in bedding, new research shows that cold water washing will eliminate 85% to 90% of the mite allergen.

Replace curtains with washable ones, or with venetian blinds. Put away any dust-collecting knickknacks, books, records and stuffed animals. Store clothing in drawers in plastic, and put out-of-season clothes in a closet away from the bedroom. And do focus on the bedroom, since that's where you spend a great deal of time. Replacing or removing bedroom carpets and drapes can make a dramatic difference.

Mite control is not particularly difficult – especially if you understand the ways of the dust mite. Look at your dust mite duty as an opportunity to redecorate, and you'll have a cleaner, fresher, happier environment. Treat what you don't replace, and give the mites fewer places to live.

Seasonal allergic rhinitis

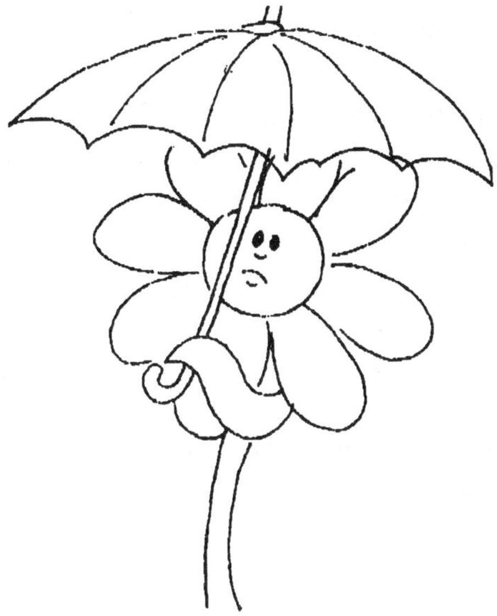

Spring is in the air, and so is pollen. Pollen and mold spores are the most common causes of seasonal allergic rhinitis, a condition which affects approximately 35 million people.

Seasonal allergies, or pollinosis, accounts for over 8.4 million trips to the doctor, annually, in the U.S. And believe it or not, allergies are the sixth leading cause of chronic illness in our country. All this just because Mother Nature wants to carry on.

Pollen

Plants depend on the wind for pollination and reproduction. The pollen is released into the air. When you're sensitive to the pollen and you breathe in the small particles, your nose becomes irritated and inflamed. You then begin to sneeze, get congested, and maybe even get itchy, watery eyes and a sore throat.

Trees, grasses, and weeds are the biggest offenders. Most flowers rely on insects for their pollination needs. They don't cause rhinitis unless a person is in very close contact with the offending flower. In the Northern and Eastern U.S., tree pollen begins to saturate the air as early as April. As the season progresses, grass pollens begin to be released.

Rose fever is a common name often applied to spring and summer allergy sufferers. Most rhinitis sufferers are not allergic to roses; it's just coincidental that they're blooming at this time.

The term "hayfever" is applied to fall allergy sufferers. Ragweed is the primary offender during this season. The ragweed season usually begins in late August and runs through September. In the U.S., 75% of all seasonal allergy sufferers are victims of ragweed. Approximately 40% are offended by grass allergies, and 9% by tree allergies. The reason the numbers add up to more than 100% is that 25% of us are lucky enough to suffer from a combination of ragweed and grass allergies. An unfortunate 5% are made miserable by all three allergens.

Mold

Airborne mold is also cause for concern by many allergy sufferers. The mold season usually begins in the early spring and peaks in the warm summer months. The first frost and the coming of cold, dry air usually marks the demise of the mold season.

Sneezing, a runny nose, and congestion are the most common and irritating symptoms. Sneezing is most likely to occur in the morning. The patient may experience a sneezing attack of upwards of 20 sneezes in rapid succession. Often, eyes will water or tear. This is caused by stimulation of the tear ducts during the sneeze.

Why Do You Sneeze?

Why do you sneeze? Well it's your body's way of blasting out something that's irritating the nose. Because the pollen is so small, and because there's so much of it, a sneeze rarely works.

By the time your body recognizes that the pollen is there, it's a little too late; the irritation has already begun. So the body resorts to another tactic: it tries to flush the irritation out.

This is where the runny nose comes in. The medical term is rhinorrhea. It's defined as a thin, watery discharge from the nose – as if someone left a faucet running in there.

The watery-looking discharge should be just that: clear and thin. If it becomes

yellow or green, there's an infection present.

Usually the discharge associated with an infection is thick and mucusy. It makes the nasal congestion worse and may contribute to headaches and earaches.

The Eustachian tubes connect your inner ear and your throat. Their purpose is to equalize the pressure behind your eardrums. They can become clogged with mucus and cause a painful earache and difficulty hearing. This can usually be alleviated by swallowing, and by using over-the-counter (OTC) decongestants.

The nasal turbinate are folds of skin, like membranes, inside your nose. The folds provide an increased surface area, which gives your nose a larger filter to clean the air you breathe. When they're irritated by pollen, they swell. That's the main cause of nasal congestion.

Diagnosis

Diagnosis of seasonal allergic rhinitis is fairly simple: you experience the symptoms and discomfort during the proper season. Confirming the diagnosis and pinpointing the allergen is another matter. Skin testing is the preferred method used by physicians. If your skin test is positive, there's little need for further testing. Alternatively, the RAST test is a lab test that can be used to confirm the diagnosis by checking for an immunologic reaction to the allergen in a blood sample.

If the skin test is negative but symptoms persist, a nasal provocation or challenge test is another method used to confirm the diagnosis.

Infectious Rhinitis

Infectious Rhinitis is the term given to rhinitis complicated by a bacterial or a viral infection. Typically, these sufferers have a fever, sore throat and swollen lymph glands in addition to the other symptoms. They also have a yellow or green discharge. Diagnosis is made by lab testing and a nasal swab. This is a long, cotton swab-like object that's used to wipe the inside of the nose. Then it's taken to the lab to be tested for specific organisms. The appropriate antibiotic can then be prescribed. These sufferers usually need help with the relief of their other symptoms, as well. Drugstore cough medicine and decongestants are often helpful.

Perennial Allergic Rhinitis is a variation of allergic rhinitis that occurs continuously, or without seasonal variation. The symptoms are the same as those of seasonal rhinitis, but usually not as severe. It's believed that this condition is the result of constant exposure to an allergen. There are cases of food allergies masquerading as perennial allergic rhinitis. Diagnosis and testing becomes very complicated.

Coping With Rhinitis

How can you cope with rhinitis? The best way is to avoid coming into contact with the allergen that offends your nose. Stay indoors as much as possible if you suffer from the seasonal variety. Vacuum with an allergy-trapping vacuum, and dust often to avoid giving dust mites an opportunity to set up housekeeping. Keep windows and doors closed. Use the air conditioner as much as possible and be sure to change the filter regularly. If you have central air, get an electrostatic or 3M Filtrete filter, and then run the system on fan (or cool or heat) for 15 minutes several times a day.

Dry your clothes with a clothes dryer instead of hanging them on a clothesline. Pollen settles on clothes that are aired outside.

A HEPA filter can also help keep the air in your bedroom clean.

Breathe through your nose as much as possible. Your nose has a natural filter system that your mouth doesn't.

If you must exercise out-of-doors, select a location that doesn't maximize your exposure to the allergens. In other words, if you're allergic to trees, don't go for a jog through the park. When selecting furnishings for your home, avoid carpets if possible. If you do select carpeting, choose a variety that has a low pile and is color-safe for frequent cleaning. Avoid down comforters and pillows and wool blankets. Opt for the synthetic, non-allergenic varieties that are available.

Of course, you can't live in a bubble. So if you're exposed, or do suffer occasional symptoms, there are some drug treatments that can work. Antihistamines in both the basic retail and the prescription varieties are the most often-used medications. Nasal anti-inflammatories are also useful for helping ease the discomfort. Your healthcare provider and your pharmacist can offer the best advice on the right drug for you. But remember, the best medicine is to avoid the allergen.

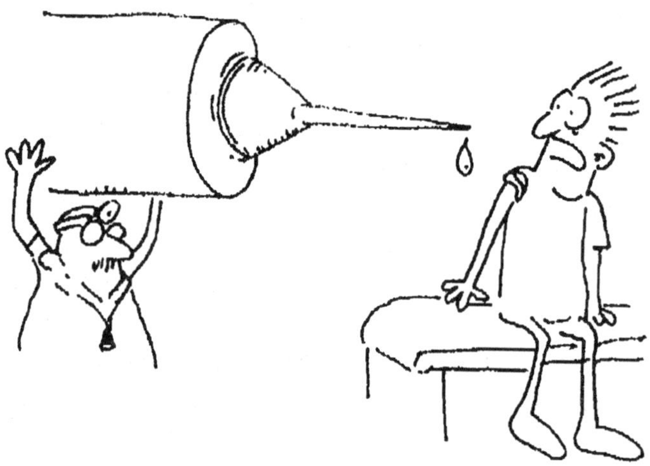

Latex allergies

Over the past decade, the FDA has received more than 1,700 reports of severe allergic reactions, including 16 deaths, related to medical devices containing latex. The deaths all occurred in 1989 among children with spina bifida, and were caused by a reaction to latex cuffs used on the tip of barium enema catheters.

FDA Requires Latex Allergy Warning

The FDA has ordered makers of all medical devices that contain latex to warn that the products may cause allergic reactions. Products covered include everything from latex surgical gloves to anesthesia equipment.

Most Americans have a low risk of an allergic reaction to latex – less than 1%, according to the FDA. People who are repeatedly exposed to latex are at increased risk, including health care workers and patients with repeat surgeries.

The new regulation requires every medical device containing latex to state that fact on the label and to carry the allergy warning, "Caution: This product contains natural rubber latex which may cause allergic reactions."

A Treatment For Latex Allergy

A treatment for latex allergy has been developed. The technique is based on a simple concept: if you put an allergen under the tongue for a few minutes, it goes into the bloodstream. This minimal exposure over time helps build up your immune system's tolerance to the antigen.

A 1996 report by Drs. Morris, Kroker, Sabnis and Morris of La Crosse, Wisconsin looked at recent double-blind, placebo-controlled studies from Europe, where sublingual treatment was effective at treating allergies to dust mites and grass.

The American doctors have also tried out sublingual treatments with patients who have history of a strong reaction to latex. They gave them latex antigens, along with other inhalant antigens, three times a day under the tongue.

They followed the patients for six months or more, and the results were excellent. The patients showed clinical improvement, decreased skin reactivity (to skin tests), and decreased levels of IgE antibodies to latex in their bloodstream. There were no adverse reactions to the treatment.

The doctors suggest that treatment of such a potent allergen as latex may also reduce cross-reactivity associated with latex allergy. People with latex allergy are usually also allergic to banana, avocado, chestnut and papain, which is used in meat tenderizer and in beer. The researchers believe that reducing the latex allergy can help reduce the problems the latex-allergic have with these foods.

The doctors concluded that sublingual treatment offers safe, effective, and specific allergy management for patients with latex allergy. *These treatments should be done under close medical supervision – don't try this at home!*

Housework can be risky!

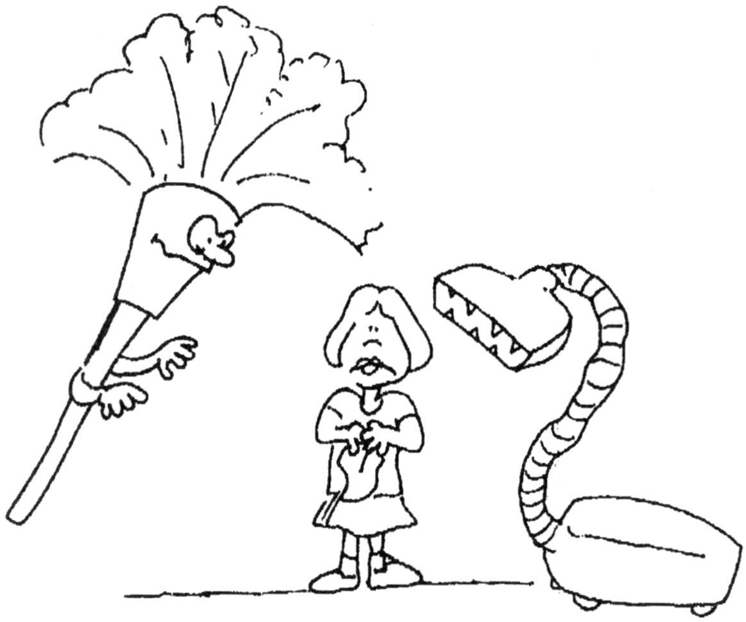

Did you ever stop to think that housework could be dangerous to your health? Because you suffer from allergies, you can attest to this. There are many hidden allergens and irritants in the average home. Let's take a look at some of them and see if your home can pass the White Glove test.

Biological Hazards

Biological hazards are the most common irritants found in American homes. These include dust mites, animal dander, bacteria and mold. All can settle or grow in overlooked nooks and crannies.

The most common household irritant is the **dust mite**. This is a lovely, microscopic creature that can be found in every home. He lives primarily in bed linens, carpets, and upholstered furniture.

In a crude sense, the dust mite's most irritating habit is that he poops everywhere. In fact, he can produce over twenty different droppings each day. These droppings are the principle component of house dust, which contains an allergen.

The dust mite isn't a completely inhospitable house guest – after all, he does clean up after himself by eating his own poop! But he then, of course, poops again. And this time, the allergen's power is multiplied.

The good news is that the little guys don't live very long. The bad news is that female dust mites can lay up to fifty eggs each, and produce a new generation every three weeks. (They're such a nuisance that we've given them their own chapter elsewhere in this book.)

Researchers recommend that, for allergy sufferers, the bedroom should be the primary area of dust mite eradication. We spend 1/3 of our life in this room and it's usually bedecked with dust mite-accommodating curtains, pillows, and blankets.

To control dust mite infestation, linens should be washed weekly. It's also recommended that carpets and heavy curtains be avoided, and that furniture and lamps be kept well-dusted.

If you have extreme dust mite allergies, you should buy special allergy-resistant zipper cases for your mattresses and pillows. A vacuum cleaner with a multi-layered bag and an exhaust filter is also helpful, as is a home HEPA filtration system. A less drastic, and far less effective tactic is to use your air conditioner. Be sure to change the filters regularly.

Animal allergens are particularly irritating to some. Cat allergen is primarily a product of the animal's skin and dried saliva. Believe it or not, you don't have to own a pet to suffer. Animal allergens are sticky, and have been found on the clothes and in the homes of people who merely visit people with pets. Contact with the allergen is rarely irritating. It's usually most offensive as an airborne irritant that's inhaled by unsuspecting sufferers. Unfiltered vacuums are prime offenders in blowing the stuff around. The allergen particles are so small that they pass through the bag's walls and out the exhaust system.

Animal allergen also has an amazing shelf life. It can be found on walls, molding and other hard surfaces up to six months after the offending animal has been banned from the room. In one study, cat allergen was found all around a house that hadn't had cats as tenants for *ten years!* To rid your house of some of that animal allergen, wipe down your walls, windows and light fixtures with a warm, soapy solution. A treatment with Allersearch X-Mite™ can denature animal allergens, as well as dust mite allergen. X-Mite is a powder that you sprinkle on carpet and upholstery (except white fabric), let sit, then vacuum up a few hours later. And it really works!

The last class of irritating household biologicals incorporates **living matter**. In our grandparents' day, standing water was a breeding ground for the mosquito which carries Yellow Fever. For us, there are other illnesses that can grow in the most unsuspecting places. We've all heard of the outbreaks of Legionnaires' Disease – usually associated with large hotels and office buildings. But residential cooling systems can also harbor the bacterium that causes this respiratory illness. Tap water and whirlpool baths have also been identified as hospitable to this creature, as well as others that cause illness.

And if you think Pontiac Fever is something you catch in the back seat of a car, you are sadly mistaken. It's really a flu-like illness similar to Legionnaires' Disease that can make you miserable for 3 to 5 days.

To combat these **bacteria**, domestic engineers recommend that water not be allowed to pool or stand for any length of time. Wiping tubs, saunas, and whirlpools out with chlorine bleach or an industrial-strength quaternium disinfectant is a good preventative.

Hantavirus is the mysterious fatal respiratory illness that befuddled medical authorities in the desert Southwest. It's a **virus** transmitted in mice and rodent droppings, which dry out and become a dust that you breathe.

Molds are by far the most offensive living biological irritant. They love warm, humid, out-of-the-way places and there are literally thousands of different varieties.

In defense of molds, it can be said that we in the medical profession owe them a lot. Penicillin is a good mold. But the chance of you growing something healthy in your kitchen exhaust fan is slim to none. The most irritating mold-like quality is the spores they emit as a means of reproduction. These are usually sent airborne by the mold in an attempt to reach another mold colony and establish their own housekeeping. Bathrooms and kitchens are the most humid rooms in the house and, therefore, natural habitats for molds.

Perhaps the best way to combat these invaders is, very simply, to open a window or use an exhaust fan. If you're remodeling, mold inhibitors can be added to some paints. There's also an electrically powered mold zapper which can be purchased. It has a heating chamber that sucks in and kills the mold spores. Though it lacks the charming zzzzzztttt sound of its cousin, the outdoor bug zapper, it works on the same principle.

Volatile Organic Compounds

Volatile Organic Compounds (VOCs) are another category of household irritants that can cause illness. These are the chemicals, solvents, powerful cleansers and insecticides that we use everyday in and around our homes. You can usually tell a VOC by its remarkably long chemical name, and the fact that it evaporates quickly (which is what is meant by "volatile"). They can cause an array of complications, depending on the chemicals involved. It's a good rule of thumb to wear gloves, open a window, and avoid mixing these chemicals while working around the house.

A common mistake is the indiscriminate mixing of chlorine bleach and ammonia products. This produces phosgene gas – a crude nerve gas used in wars earlier this century. It overcomes the user and can be fatal. More and more brand name products contain either chlorine or ammonia – so be careful!

It's also a good idea to keep the telephone number of the nearest poison control center in a handy place when using chemicals and, of course, the easiest prevention is to always read the label and not mix products!

Other Household Irritants

The final category of potential household health irritants is airborne heavy metals and gases. We all know the hazard **lead** paint can present to small children if they eat it. But did you know that if it's not stripped properly (such as when you're renovating your house) it can become airborne? Inhaling lead paint dust can cause some horrible health problems!

Lead is also a component in some arts and crafts like stained glass-making. Some of that lead can go airborne, too.

Latex paint isn't completely safe, either. Some of these products contain phenylmercuric acid (PMA), which emits mercury vapor and can cause mercury poisoning. (Remember the Mad Hatter from Alice in Wonderland? He suffered from mercury poisoning – a common ailment for hatters who used mercury fumes to shape the hat.)

And, of course, airborne **asbestos** fiber is a hazard in many older homes, too.

The gas that has gotten the most press in the last few years is **radon**. As uranium decays, it becomes radium. That, in turn, becomes radon, a gas that gives off radioactive alpha particles as it further breaks down. These particles are odorless, tasteless and colorless. They are reported to be the second leading cause of lung cancer. There are radon test kits and treatment kits available in hardware and household stores.

It's interesting to note that **smoking** (the leading cause of lung cancer) and radon exposure both compound the risk of lung cancer. Studies suggest that smokers have a 20 times higher risk of developing lung cancer when exposed to radon than nonsmokers.

In review, keeping a house is a risky business. As America becomes more health-conscious, there are builders who are constructing environmentally-safe and hypoallergenic homes. These are homes that are constructed with untreated, naturally processed materials and have innovations that make them more environmentally friendly. Internal HEPA filtration systems, water filters, and specially designed heating and cooling systems are among the many innovations being incorporated.

If you can't afford a new house, your old one can be modified and upgraded. With a little common sense and attention to cleaning technique, your home can become allergy-free. Or you can join the millions of people (like me!) who have decided that housework is just too darn dangerous to our health and well-being.

Part 4
Medications

Medication Basics

The way we think about medications for the treatment of asthma is changing. There are two reasons behind this. The first reason for the change in thought is that medical science has redefined asthma. It's now thought of as a *chronic* illness with *two components*: an inflammatory one, and a restrictive one.

Because of this, we now use medications to tackle asthma from both the inflammatory and the restrictive angles.

The addition of the word *chronic* also radically changes the approach. Chronic means the illness develops slowly and lasts a long time – even a lifetime. So the medical world is finally acknowledging that asthma is a long-term problem.

Based on the concept that asthma is a chronic disease, The National Heart, Blood and Lung Institute is now recommending long-term treatment programs. Treatment has been divided into two paths, prevention and emergency relief.

The current thinking is that it's better to prevent an asthma attack by interrupting the mechanism that triggers it, than it is to try and stop one that has already started. Researchers are now searching for medications that inhibit the body's responses, rather than correct them. Specifically, medications are being reclassified as controllers and relievers.

Controllers are medications that are taken to repress the asthmatic tendency. They are taken for long-term management. The purpose of these medications is to prevent the symptoms of airflow limitation caused by both the inflammation and the restriction so common in an asthma attack. These drugs may include long-lasting bronchodilators and anti-inflammatories. They also include corticosteroids, as well as anti-allergic agents.

Relievers are medications that are short-acting and help interrupt and relieve the immediate symptoms of an asthma attack. A good way to think of reliever medications is as your emergency medications. These medications are primarily Beta agonists of the bronchodilator category.

The way you take each of these medications has a dramatic effect on the way they work and the benefit you receive from them.

Taking medication by mouth in either pill or liquid form is good for long term or controller type therapies. The drug is taken into your body through the natural processes of digestion. The medication usually takes longer to enter your system, and as a rule, the effects last a little longer. The down side to taking medication this way is that it circulates throughout your body through your bloodstream. This means that all of your body is exposed to the medication. That increases the likelihood that you'll have a reaction to the medication. It also means that more medication is required to treat your asthma, since some of it goes to waste circulating around in your blood, going to parts of your body that don't need it.

Inhaling or breathing in medication is a good alternative to taking it by mouth. This way, more of the medication goes directly to the lungs and the sites where it's needed most. This drug isn't wasted in the blood system, so the response is quicker and less drug is usually required. Also, because it's being used up at the location where it's most needed, less of the drug is absorbed into your body. Thus, the likelihood of having a reaction is greatly diminished. These are the main reasons the inhaled method is now the preferred method of giving asthma medication.

Aerosolizing or nebulizing the medication is a process in which the drug is placed in a chamber and a gas passes through it, turning it into a fine mist. You then breathe the mist in either through a mouthpiece or a mask. This is the treatment that most asthmatics receive in the Emergency Room when they're having an attack.

Many asthmatics have home nebulizer machines. They buy their medications in either pre-mixed unit dose vials or they use a bottle with an eye dropper and add normal saline. Normal saline is water with a little salt in it. It's manufactured to be just the amount of salt that matches your body's salt level. Remember how salty your tears taste? Normal saline has that same taste. It's important that if you're ever called upon to give yourself a treatment, that you always use normal saline, and never plain water. Water is very irritating to your lungs. It will cause you to cough violently and may make your asthma attack worse. We've all inhaled water accidentally while swimming. Remember how irritating and uncomfortable that was? In addition to home nebulizer systems, there are many portable, handheld models for people on the go. They are battery operated.

An ultrasonic nebulizer is similar to a standard nebulizer, but it puts out a finer mist, with smaller-sized particles. Think of the difference between the two as the same as a fine rain, compared to a hard rain with big drops. Like the conventional nebulizer, there are both home and portable models. Both also require a physician's order.

An ultrasonic nebulizer can be preferable if you have a problem getting mucus out of your lungs. The finer mist goes deeper into the lungs and adds more moisture. In essence, it wets the lungs more quickly and helps break up that mucus.

If you don't need the ultrasonic nebulizer to help get the secretions out ... then you're just putting more moisture into your lungs that you'll have to cough out.

Metered Dose Inhalers (MDI) are the most common delivery system for asthma medications. You probably have one in your pocket or purse right now. It's the little pump sprayer which puts out an exact amount of medicine, which you breathe in.

The most effective way to use these inhalers is with a spacer device or a holding chamber. That's a tube-like plastic thing that you spray the inhaler into before breathing the medication in. The benefit of using the spacer is that more of the medication goes directly into your lungs. Here's why: If you place the inhaler directly into your mouth and spray, a large part of the medication ends up in your mouth and around your teeth and gums. Obviously, it doesn't do much good there. The spacer allows more of the medication to get where it's needed most – your lungs.

There are several other devices to help you use your MDI more efficiently. If you have trouble activating or squeezing your MDI, there are various assistance aids. There's even an electronic one that squeezes for you and keeps count of how many you have taken and the time you took them. You simply push a button and it delivers a puff.

Properly using your MDI and spacer is easy. Take the canister out of the plastic holder. Place it in the spacer device. Shake the canister vigorously for one to two minutes. Take a few deep breaths while you are shaking. Exhale completely and place the mouthpiece of the spacer in your mouth. Breathe in deeply, activating the canister as you do so. Hold your breath for a count of ten and exhale.

If you have to take a second puff, wait a few minutes and then repeat the process. If you are using two different inhalers, wait a few minutes between each. Give your lungs a chance to absorb the first one and then take the second. This helps your body use both medications effectively.

You may want to rinse your mouth out after you take your MDI. This will remove the excess medication that does get deposited in your mouth, and takes away the bad taste that some medications have. Wash your spacer in warm soapy water and rinse it thoroughly every day.

Keeping track of how many puffs you have taken from a canister is perhaps the biggest problem most MDI users report. They don't know when the canister is empty. Sadly, the MDI will continue to spray long after the medication has run out. You think you're getting a dose of medicine, but you're really only receiving the propellant that's left in the canister.

There's an easy way to test the canisters and tell if they're used up. Simply remove the canister from the holder and place it in a bowl of water. If it floats, it's empty. If it sinks, it's full. A half full canister will bob up and down like a buoy. This is a simple and accurate check which most pharmacists don't have the time to teach

How full is your MDI canister? Place it in a bowl of water to find out!

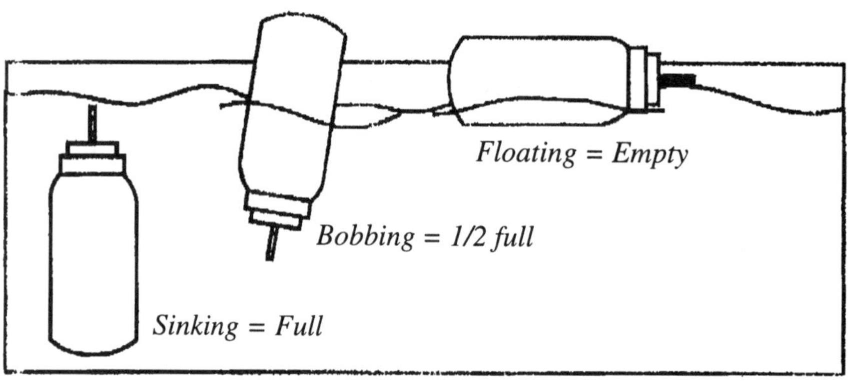

and most physicians don't know. It's a good idea to test your MDI every few days and to refill your prescription when there is 1/4 left in the canister. That way you won't run out of medication.

MDI therapy has been proven effective for children, too. Most spacer devices have a mask attachment for toddlers and specific instructions on the best way to use them. During acute or severe asthma attacks, it's difficult for most kids to use MDI's. A nebulizer with a mask is probably a better choice to insure the medication is getting in.

The MDI industry as we know it is in a little trouble. Because of the damage to the ozone layer caused by chlorofluorocarbons (CFCs), many manufacturers have to reformulate their products. Many MDI's use CFCs as their principal propellant. The Montreal Agreement bans the production and use of CFCs. But an exemption for MDIs and medically necessary treatments has been requested. An extension has been granted and it is expected that a permanent exemption will be approved. So don't worry. While your MDI may be changing in the next few years, you'll still be able to get your medication in the same handy format.

Researchers are developing alternative hand-held delivery devices that don't depend on CFCs. Breath-activated inhalers are one alternative, and dry powder inhalers are another. Many of these new alternatives are being introduced in the U.S. Because each drug manufacturer is working on their own type of dry inhaler, you'll need to ask your pharmacist and even call the company for directions. Many have videos and booklets that explain how to use the new inhalers.

Medication is an integral and vital part of asthma management. The type of medication you take, as well as how you take it, has a direct impact on your asthma symptoms. When in doubt, ask your health care provider what's best for you, and make sure all your questions get answered.

How to use a spacer device

A spacer device is a round plastic tube that acts as a holding chamber for your medication. It helps you coordinate the timing of your medication and deliver the most medication to your lungs where it is needed. When you use your MDI (metered dose inhaler) without a spacer device, a lot of the medication ends up in your mouth and goes to waste. A good rule of thumb is: If you can taste the medication, you aren't taking it properly.

How To Use a Spacer Device

1. First, remove the metal medication canister from the plastic holder.
2. Remove the cap from the spacer device and place the stem of the metal canister in the spacer device.
3. Shake the medication canister and the spacer device for at least one minute.
4. Exhale completely.
5. Place the mouthpiece of the spacer device in your mouth and breathe in.
6. Squeeze down on the canister of medication as you breathe in. (If it's hard for you to squeeze and breathe at the same time, you can place the spacer in your mouth, squeeze down on the canister, and then breathe in. The first method is better, but this works, too.)
7. Remove the spacer from your mouth and hold your breath for a count of ten.
8. If your physician has ordered you to take two puffs of your medication, wait a few minutes and then take the second puff just as you did the first.
9. If you're taking two different types of medications you can use the same spacer device. Just wait a few minutes between each.
10. It's a good idea to wash your spacer device with warm, soapy water on a regular basis. Be sure to dry it well.

Drugs for allergies, asthma and pulmonary problems

In this section, we'll get into specifics about asthma drugs, plus take a look at drugs for allergy sufferers and pulmonary patients. We're going to focus on five specific categories of medications. It's important that you understand each, and when and if you should take them.

When determining the medication you should take, it's important to suit the action of the medication to the specific problem you're experiencing. This sounds like common sense, but most people really don't know which medication has what effect. Then they don't take the right medication at the right time.

The first two categories, relievers and controllers, are very important for asthma sufferers. Drugs of the third category, antihistamines, are used frequently by allergy sufferers. The next two categories, mucolytics and expectorants, may be used, from time to time, by people with all types of respiratory problems. The fifth category includes some over-the-counter medications. The sixth category is herbal remedies.

Airway Relievers

Airway relievers are short-acting medications that relieve or slow down the contraction of your airway. Asthma is characterized by bronchial restriction and by inflammation. During an attack your airway tightens up and it feels as if you're breathing through a straw. Making matters worse, inflammation kicks in and mucus plugs up the straw.

Relievers work to open the airway up so the straw is more like a garden hose. Many other patients besides asthma sufferers take relievers. People with emphysema, chronic bronchitis or bronchiectasis (destruction of the bronchial walls) are also given these medications to help ease their breathing.

The medications most often classified as relievers are a class of drugs known as short-acting beta agonists. These can be taken as a liquid or pill, or breathed into the lungs through a nebulizer, metered dose inhaler (MDI), or a non-pressurized inhaler.

The effects of a reliever medication usually last about four hours. You can take it at periodic intervals and as an emergency helper when you begin to feel that you're having difficulty. Your physician can best help you decide which time-schedule is best for you.

Many people take relievers with a home nebulizer. If this is the route you generally use, you should also have an MDI to carry with you in your purse or pocket, in case you aren't home when you're due for a treatment.

Some physicians believe having an MDI of the same medication is an added expense to the patient or that it's an opportunity for the patient to overuse the medication. We think it makes a lot of sense, as it gives you the freedom to leave home for longer periods without having to stop at the emergency room on your way back.

Before we go much further, let's explain why these medications are relievers. Your body has three types of receptors: alpha, beta 1 and beta 2. Receptors are places on the surface of a cell where an antigen lands and locks in to produce an immunologic component. It's like a key fitting into a lock – only certain keys will fit certain locks. When the lock is opened, the allergic consequences (good or bad) start to unfold.

Alpha receptors are found in your airways, in your blood vessels and in your heart. Stimulating your alpha receptors may ease your bronchial constriction, but it will also make your heart beat faster and cause your blood pressure to increase.

Beta 1 receptors are not found in the muscles of your airways but are in the blood vessels of the airways and in the heart. Stimulating them also causes your heart rate to go up.

Beta 2 receptors are located in the muscle tissue of your airways and a few are found in the heart. These are the receptors we try most often to use when dealing with asthma or pulmonary conditions.

In the early days of asthma therapy, we didn't know about all the receptor sites and what they did. One of the first things researchers learned is that our bodies naturally produce two chemicals: epinephrine and norepinephrine, both of which are neurotransmitters that send a message to constrict blood flow through vasoconstriction, or narrowing the blood vessels.

Epinephrine is produced by the adrenal gland and causes smooth muscle contraction. This occurs when the *alpha* receptors in the muscle tissue are stimulated by the drug.

Norepinephrine is produced by the nerve endings. This hormone works on the *beta* receptors and results in smooth muscle relaxation.

Bronchial constriction is a problem for both allergy and asthma sufferers, and both alpha and beta receptors are found in the bronchial tissue. In treating bronchial constriction, the goal is to stimulate just the beta receptors. To do this, researchers have tried for the better part of this century to develop beta-selective medications. Their work has formed the basis for the way we treat bronchoconstriction.

In both asthma and allergy sufferers, we use *beta agonists*, and particularly short-acting ones, as relievers. An agonist is a drug which has an affinity for a specific cell type – or receptor – and which produces a predictable response. An *antagonist* would be a substance which competes for the same receptor site, but which has an opposite response. Beta agonists are also called beta adrenergics or beta-adrenergic receptor agonists.

What are the side effects of short-acting beta agonists? While each medication has its specific effects, there are some general side effects you should be aware of. They can make your heart beat a little faster and your hands tingle. They can cause nausea, headache, and a feeling of anxiousness or restlessness.

If you experience any of these symptoms you should discuss them with your physician. It may mean your dosage needs adjusting, or perhaps there's a better medication for you.

The side effect that most physicians and pharmacists forget to tell you about is rebound. This is traditionally associated with overuse of a medication. It can occur as a result of high dosages or long-term use of the medication. Rebound is like stretching a rubber band. If you put all five of your fingers inside a rubber band and stretch it, it opens up. But when you take your fingers out it snaps back. That's what your airway does. Instead of being stretched by the medication, it snaps back even tighter and narrower, making it hard for you to breathe.

An example of rebound is found with some of the over-the-counter nasal decongestants, particularly inhalers for clearing sinuses. They work fine at first, but as the dose wears off, the congestion worsens – often to the point where it's worse than before you used the decongestant.

Drugs in the short-acting beta agonist category include:

Albuterol (Proventil, Ventolin) is probably the most widely-used reliever medication. Albuterol sulfate was introduced in 1968 and is today the most popular beta agonist in the U.S. It's available in many forms, including oral, syrup, MDI, IV, aerosol, and a drug powder for spin inhalers.

Side effects include heart problems (especially for the tablets) and tremors (more likely with the inhaled versions.)

Albuterol is used extensively throughout Europe as an intravenous medication. But it's not approved for that use in the U.S. In Europe the medication is known as Salbutamol.

Epinephrine, a synthetic version of the natural compound the body produces, was first used in the early part of this century to relieve asthma symptoms. It's a potent alpha adrenergic stimulator, and non-selective beta adrenergic stimulator. It stimulates both the beta 1 and beta 2 receptors. In essence, it stimulates everything without much selectivity. It can be given by injection or by aerosolization.

Epinephrine's side effects include tachycardia (rapid heart rate), nervousness, palpitations, tachyarrythmias (rapid, irregular heart rate), headache, tremor, and systemic hypertension. It should be used with caution in people who have cardiac disease and hyperthyroidism. The systemic (system-wide) side effects are reduced when given by aerosol. MDI preparations are available.

Epinephrine is still widely used in instances of severe, acute asthma, usually by physicians in the emergency room. It has a shorter duration of action than many other medications and is rapidly metabolized, or used up, by our bodies.

Many allergy sufferers are familiar with epinephrine because it's used during severe allergic reactions, including anaphylactic shock. Depending on the severity of the reaction you're having, the dosage and the way the physician administers this medication may vary. Generally, the more rapidly it gets into your blood system, the stronger the effect epi will have. An injection straight into your vein will work faster and be more potent than a shot just under the skin (subcutaneous).

But there are a few points to consider. The shot in the vein will work faster and will also be used up faster, which means you may need more. It will also have a direct impact on your heart, which may not be a good thing. These are points the doctor will weigh. These decisions must be made by a person with training and experience using this medication (in other words, don't try this at home. But if you are prone to anaphylactic reactions, you can get an EpiPen and the education to safely give yourself an emergency epinephrine shot.)

Isoproterenol hydrochloride (Isuprel) has gradually replaced epinephrine in the U.S. This drug has less of an alpha response than epinephrine. It's usually given as a nebulizer treatment. It can also be given as a pill under the tongue, but this is not the most effective way to take it. Isoproterenol can also be given to asthma patients through an IV. This is not recommended for adults due to some limited cardiac side effects. It's available in both MDI and aerosol forms. Like epinephrine, isoproterenol is quickly metabolized and thus short-acting, rapidly relaxing the bronchial muscles and then passing on through the system.

Isoetharine (Bronkosol) was introduced to the U.S. in 1951. It offers rapid relief, with activity lasting between one and three hours. Isoetharine is a considerable improvement over the short duration of isoproterenol and epinephrine. In the U.S., isoetharine is available in MDI and aerosol forms. Elsewhere in the world, the oral form is preferred.

Metaproterenol (Alupent) was introduced to the U.S. in 1961. It's a derivative of isoproterenol that has a longer duration of action and fewer side effects. When taken orally, it begins to work in 30 minutes, and continues for up to five hours. It's also available in aerosol and MDI form.

Terbutaline (Bricanyl, Brethine, Brethaire) is a first-generation engineered beta-adrenergic receptor agonist. It's available in an MDI, and is also given orally or by subcutaneous injection. It's often given by aerosol, too, although this route has not been approved in the U.S. This medication is a potent relaxer of the smooth muscle cells. Because of this, it's also used to halt premature contractions during pregnancy. The bad news is that it tends to have a few more side effects than the other drugs we've talked about.

Short-acting beta agonists are frequently used in combination with other drugs to maximize effectiveness and control bronchial constriction. They are most often taken in association with medications like **theophylline** (Theo-Dur, Slo-Bid, Uniphyl) and its derivative **aminophylline**. These medications relieve bronchoconstriction via a different route, and they take a little longer to work. Studies suggest that when taken together, theophylline and a beta agonist complement each other.

The oral route is the preferred method because it's the easiest and most cost-effective. If given the option, it's recommended that separate pills be taken, as opposed to a combined form. This provides the most flexibility for the patient and regularity of dosage. Short-acting beta agonists are also combined with the next class of drugs we'll talk about: controllers, or long-acting beta agonists.

Controllers

Controllers are medications that play a key role in preventing asthma attacks from happening. They are either long-acting beta adrenergic agonists that control bronchial constriction over long periods of time (8 to 12 hours or longer), or they are medications that control the inflammatory part of asthma and prevent it from happening. Let's take a look at the long-acting beta-adrenergic agonists first.

Salmeterol (Serevent®) is one of the newest of the long-acting beta-adrenergic agonists. It's chemically similar to albuterol, but offers a longer period of action. In fact, this medication can last up to 12 hours in cases of moderate asthma, and even longer in mild asthmatic conditions. It's believed to have some anti-inflammatory effects as well, but is usually given along with steroids.

Salmeterol is removed from your body by your liver and should be used with caution by patients with liver and heart difficulties.

Pirbuterol acetate (Maxair) is available in both MDI and a breathing-activated inhaler unit (free of CFCs). This medication is similar to albuterol, but has a slower onset and longer bronchodilator effects.

Bitolterol (Tornalate) was developed here in the U.S. It's known as a pro-drug which means that it's a chemical which your body converts into another drug, in this case, colterol. Because your body needs to convert it, it's not a very rapidly-acting drug. Similar to the short-acting terbutaline, its effects last 6 to 8 hours.

Fenoterol is a potent bronchodilator that may have received a bad rap in the media. It was reported in association with a series of deaths in Australia. There are differing opinions as to whether or not the medication was the cause, if it was misused. It's not presently available in the U.S.

Formoterol is another long-acting beta agonist being used in Europe. It's not presently available in the U.S, but will probably be available here shortly.

Corticosteroids are the next type of controller medications we will examine. These are frequently combined with beta agonists (both long-acting and short-acting) to control asthmatic symptoms. They work by inhibiting or slowing down the inflammation process, making them powerful anti-inflammatories.

Since each of the steroids works a little differently, the exact effect they have on your body may be different, too. If you're taking a corticosteroid, learn more about that specific one.

The short-term side effects associated with corticosteroids include a dry mouth, weight gain, high blood pressure, yeast infections, hoarseness, and coughing. These medications can be taken by either nebulizer, inhaler, pill, or IV. Oral doses of these medications have been linked to delayed growth in children, and the development of osteoporosis, diabetes, ulcers, and cataracts. Generally speaking, these effects usually occur when the individual is on a high or sustained dose for a long period of time.

These medications can be delivered on a schedule (one dose every other day) or a tapering dose (smaller dose each day) to minimize the risk of side effects.

Steroids should never be stopped cold turkey! This can be potentially dangerous. They should always be gradually reduced over time until the body is weaned from their effects. This is especially true with systemic corticosteroids (taken as a pill), which can suppress the function of the hypothalamus, pituitary gland, and adrenal gland for a number of months after you stop taking them. Your doctor should be extra-vigilant if switching you to an inhaled steroid after you've been taking steroid pills. You may experience withdrawal symptoms such as joint and/or muscular pain, lassitude and depression.

It's possible to get a systemic level of steroids from the inhaled corticosteroids. The nasty effects of that include weight gain, mental disturbances, increased bruising and cataracts. In that case, discontinue use – slowly.

Dexamethasone (Decadron) was the first corticosteroid available in the U.S. as an inhaler. It's still widely used, but is losing ground to newer medications that do not require as high a dosage or have fewer side effects.

Beclomethasone (Beclovent, Beconase, Vancenase, Vanceril) is one of the newer steroids.

It's available in an MDI format. It's thought that up to 2 mg a day may be used without serious side effects. Larger doses are used in Europe. If you're on prednisone (another steroid) for other reasons, *and* take beclomethasone on alternate days, you're *more likely* to have the hypothalamus, pituitary and adrenal (HPA) problems than if you were on one drug *or* the other.

Trimcinalone (Azmacort) is another one of the new steroids. It's available as an inhaler and also in a stronger dosage as a weekly injection.

Flunisolide (Aerobid) has a longer action than some of the other medications and has recently been introduced in a mint flavor to counter patient complaints of bad taste.

Prednisone (Panasol, Prednicen-M) is one of the older corticosteroids. It comes in pill form and IV form. Cushingism is the primary concern of prednisone and related compound usage. This is a syndrome in which patients experience fatigue, weakness, weight gain, and excessive hair growth, among other symptoms.

Methylprednisolone (Solu-Medrol) is a derivative of prednisone that has slightly fewer side effects. It's usually given as an IV.

Budesonide (Rhinocort, Pulmicort Turbuhaler) is one of the newest of the steroids. It's been used in Europe for some years, and has recently become available in the U.S. It has fewer side effects than the other steroids. It's available in a nasal spray variety for allergy sufferers, as well as an inhaler for asthmatics.

Non-Steroidal Anti-Inflammatory Drugs (NSAIDs) can help asthma and allergy sufferers. Because they don't have the negative side effects of steroids, these next two are often used for children.

Cromolyn Sodium (Intal, Nasalcrom) is a mast cell stabilizer which works to fight allergies. It's also an antiasthmatic which reduces bronchial hypersensitivity. The inhaled version should be used 10 to 15 minutes *ahead* of your encountering an asthmatic trigger. It can be dangerous, though, if you use it *during* an asthma attack, with a severe anaphalyactic reaction the result.

Since it reduces the amount of histamine released, cromolyn sodium is also great for *preventing* (not treating) allergy symptoms. It contains no steroids.

Nedocromil Sodium (Tilade) is another inhaled anti-inflammatory for the prevention of asthma. It works by inhibiting the action of different types of inflammatory cells.The biggest side effect reported is a bad taste. Proper MDI use is critical.

Anticholinergic Medications reduce spasms in the bronchi by blocking the acetylcholine receptors in the parasympathetic nervous system. This part of the nervous system slows heart rate, increases movement of the intestinal tract and increases gland activity. Beta agonists, on the other hand, are *sympathomimetics*, working in the sympathetic nervous system, which speeds heart rate, constricts blood vessels and raises blood pressure.

Ipratropium Bromide (Atrovent®) is the most commonly-used anticholinergic medicine for bronchospasm. It's available as an inhaler, and in liquid form for nebulization.

Leukotreine Receptor Antagonists are a new class of medications for asthma and allergy sufferers. They went on sale in the U.S. in 1996 and we've been inundated with TV and print ads promoting these products. They work by blocking leukotrienes, which are a key part of the inflammatory process involved in early-phase and late-phase asthma. That means they stop the inflammation from happening.

The side effects of these medications include nausea, headaches, and increased risk of infections. It's recommended they be used with caution by people with liver problems.

Zafirlukast (Accolate) is one brand of leukotriene antagonist for asthma. It comes in pill form and is taken twice a day. It should be taken either one hour before, or two hours after a meal (which actually cuts the bioavailability to your body by about 40%). Always take it only when you don't have any asthma symptoms – it's not designed to reverse your bronchial spasms, but to prevent them.

Zafirlukast works by competing for the receptors used by leukotriene D_4 and E_4 (LTD_4 and LTE_4). These leukotrienes are involved with asthma symptoms such as swelling of the airway, constriction of the smooth muscle, and cellular activity associated with the inflammation process of asthma. (Asthmatics have been found to be 25 to 100 times more sensitive than non-asthmatics to the bronchoconstricting activity of LTD_4.)

In one study, it was found that taking a single dose of zafirlukast before exposure to inhaled antigens like grass, cat dander, and ragweed prevented asthma attacks.

Zafirlukast is rapidly absorbed, taking about 3 hours to reach its peak, and passing through you in 10 hours.

Drug interaction studies showed that asthma drug theophylline reduced the amount of zafirlukast in the blood by about 30%, while the theophylline level remained steady. Erithromycin reduced the availability of zafirlukast by about 40%. On the other hand, 650 mg of aspirin (4 times a day) *increased* the amount of zafirlukast in the blood by about 45%. Zafirlukast had no impact on oral contraceptives.

According to studies with over 4000 people, 12.7% reported a headache when taking zafirlukast, compared to 11.7% of those taking a placebo. That was the most commonly reported adverse effect. Some patients, particularly those over 55 who were also taking inhaled corticosteroids, reported an increase in infections. These were mostly respiratory infections.

Zileuton (Zyflo) is another new leukotriene antagonist. It's usually taken daily as a pill.

Antihistamines

Antihistamines are medications that stop the histamine response. Histamines are substances in your body that are produced from amino acids when a cell is injured. They cause the redness that occurs when you have a mosquito bite or a burn. When histamines are blocked or stopped from being released, the redness doesn't occur. For allergy sufferers, the allergic response, or runny nose, swelling and itchiness is stopped along with the histamine.

It's a fine line to walk between antihistamines and anti-inflammatory. Steroids, Cromolyn Sodium (Intal, Nasalcrom) and Nedocromil Sodium (Tilade), as well as the leukotriene antagonists could all be considered antihistamines by their activity. For the purpose of this discussion, we'll just look at the most common antihistamines.

What's the down side to antihistamines? They can cause drowsiness, dizziness, confusion, and restlessness. They can also cause nightmares. They can have some serious drug interactions. Antihistamines should be used with caution when taking digitalis, beta blockers (for the heart, not the beta agonists we talked about earlier), or MAO inhibitors. If you're taking these medications now, it doesn't mean that you can never take an antihistamine. Instead, be sure to discuss it with your physician.

If your child is taking Methylphenidate (Ritalin), you should check with your doctor before taking an antihistamine.

Diphenhydramine hydrochloride (Benadryl®) is perhaps the most common antihistamine. Discovered in the 1940s by a Florida veterinarian (who told us Parke Davis took the idea without paying him), it's now available in both prescription and non-prescription form, as well as generics. It comes in liquid, tablets or injections.

This is one product with plenty of positives and negatives. It's a versatile antihistamine, with a long list of uses, but one which also has a long list of potential side effects. (Drowsiness is the biggest one, and alcohol makes it worse.) It's used along with epinephrine to stop anaphylactic responses, yet one of the potential side effects is anaphylactic shock. It's considered an antiasthmatic/broncodilator, yet it also carries a warning for people with a history of lower respiratory disease, including asthma.

This antihistamine is good for all kinds of allergic problems, including food reactions, mild skin reactions, and even motion sickness. You can also get this medicine in a gel form for use on insect bites.

Other older antihistamines include **Atara**, **Chlortrimeton**, and 90 other products.

Recent additions to the arsenal include **Seldane** (no longer available due to interactions with erithromycin), **Tavist**, **Terfenadine**, **Hismanal**, **Allegra**, **Astemisole**, **Ceterizine**, **Loratidine**, **Trinalin**, and **Zyrtec**.

The newest of the new include **Azelastine**, **Ebastine**, **Ketotifen**, **Levocobastine**, **Mequitazine**, **Nober-astine**, **Oxatomide** and **Pemirolast**.

As you can see, the antihistamine market is big and profitable, and quite competitive. Each of the pharmaceutical companies is working hard to develop new and different antihistamines which relieve allergy symptoms without the side effects. Our recommendation is to keep nagging your doctor or allergist for different ones until you find one that works just right for you. Then, don't stick with it for too long. Switch off to another product, and use it for a while before you return to the first.

Mucolytics and Expectorants

Mucolytics help break up mucus congestion in your lungs and help your body get the secretion out. The best mucolytic agent in the world is water. Drinking plenty of water and staying well-hydrated is your body's best defense and keeps things running smoothly.

Acetylcystein (Mucomyst) is a drug that may be recommended by your doctor to help you with breaking up the mucus. If you've ever used this drug you'd remember it. It has a rotten egg smell. It comes in a liquid form and is usually nebulized. If you do happen to have it for use at home, take care when handling it. It can stain clothing and cause mild irritation to skin.

Expectorants also help you break up the secretions and cough them up. These are usually bought as over-the-counter medications and include one of two drugs: **potassium iodide** (SSKI) or **guaifenesin** (Robitussin, Muco-Fen, Humibid, Mucobid, Fenesin).

The problem with many of the expectorants is that it's tough to find them alone – they're usually sold as part of a mixture of several medications that may include an antihistamine and a cough suppressant (such as the habit-forming hydrocodone or codeine). Some of these mixtures also contain alcohol. The best bet is to read the labels carefully, or, if money isn't an issue, ask your doctor to prescribe the mixture that's exactly what you need. Remember, though, that you can usually save money buying these products at the discount store – again, read labels so you know what you're getting.

Decongestants, Cough Suppressants, and Cold Formulas

You'll find a wide array of decongestants, cough suppressants and cold formulas lining the shelves at your local drugstore. The products you see can consist of any kind of mixture the manufacturer can come up with. Many include aspirin or aspirin-substitutes, which you probably don't need.

Their side effects vary depending on the mixture. The danger of these medications is that they are easily overused and can conflict with prescriptions you're already taking. For example, you may be taking medication to lower your blood pressure and the cold formula may actually raise it. Or it could lower it to a dangerous level. The safest way to use these medications is to discuss them first with your doctor or pharmacist and know each ingredient in the mix you are planning to take. Caution should also be used because some forms of these medications may be addictive.

Pseudoephedrine hydrochloride (Sudafed®) is an over-the-counter decongestant. There are prescription combination forms that include a mix with an antihistamine. The D in the name usually refers to a decongestant, and the one of choice is pseudoephedrine hydrochloride. In some of these medications, the antihistamine is good for 12 or 24 hours, while the decongestant only works for the first three or four hours.

An example of this kind of combination is loratadine and pseudoephedrine, together as Claritin D, a 24-hour reliever.

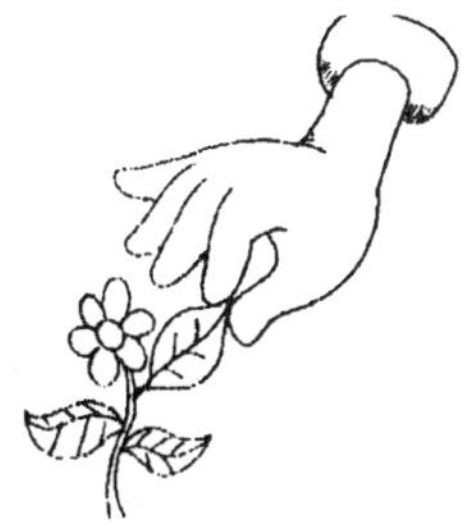

Herbal and Holistic Medications

Sometimes the things you find in the health food store are wonderful and miles ahead of what your pharmacist can offer. Other times the herbal or holistic remedies are trash. And still other products are the same as you'd find at the drug store, but under a different name.

The problem is figuring out what you're getting, and then figuring out whether it's going to work for you.

It's true that many of today's pharmaceuticals are derived from plants and herbs. One of the beautiful things about our system of for-profit drug development, though, is that an emphasis is made on focusing in on the active ingredients for the task at hand, and eliminating everything else. Purity and consistent dosage are the other hallmarks of the pharmaceutical business, and those are often difficult to find at the health food store. The other things you won't find there are scientific testing which proves safety and efficacy, or government regulation, since the new laws pretty much allow the "nutritional" businesses to say whatever they please.

So, you're ultimately left with choices. If you choose to go the alternative way, realize that the amount of information available is limited and quite questionable in its honesty and accuracy. While it's true that many herbs have been used for centuries in other cultures, that doesn't make them safe *or* effective.

Consulting a knowledgeable holistic specialist before you use these products is the safest way to go. Read books, too.

And remember that "natural" doesn't always equal safe. Some people are allergic to echinacea, and there have been anaphylactic reactions reported.

Ephedra causes the release of norepinephrine from the storage sites in the nerve endings and is a weak bronchodilator – but at high doses can have side effects such as nervousness, anxiety, insomnia, hypertension, palpitations, and tremors.

Chinese skullcap is an anti-inflammatory and an antioxidant. Some say the flavonoids in it mean that it works like Cromolyn sodium. It's available in pill form.

Green tea contains both antioxidants and theophylline-like compounds. It's believed to be a mild bronchodilator.

Caffeine also has theophylline-like compounds and has a mild bronchodilator effect. It was used for the treatment of asthma during the 1920's. So, yes, it can help relieve mild bronchospasms, but it also can have significant cardiac side effects including increased heart rate, palpitations, anxiety, hypertension, and insomnia.

Licorice root has been found to have anti-inflammatory and anti-allergic effects. But because it also has mineralocorticoid and glucocorticoid effects, it can increase the duration and strength of the effects of cortisone. It's available in tea and pill form. Don't take licorice with steroids.

Vitamin C is an anti-inflammatory, and believed to help prevent asthma attacks.

Capsicum is a found in hot peppers. It's believed to assist in relieving bronchospasms. It may also have some anti-inflammatory effects because it contains compounds similar to guaifenesin. It's available in pill or capsule form.

Garlic is a potent natural antibiotic and anti-inflammatory. It's believed that allicin is the active compound in garlic that gives it its kick. It's available in liquid, pill, and capsule form.

Skunk Cabbage is an expectorant and a sedative. It should be used with care.

Horseradish and **hot mustard** are supposed to assist in the mobilization of secretions. The belief is that the same thing that makes your eyes water and your nose run also makes your airways water (so to speak). That should make it easier for you to loosen the secretions and cough them out.

Onions are believed to be both anti-inflammatories and antibiotics. A compound known as quercetin, an antioxidant, is believed to play an antihistamine role.

Fish oil and **Omega-3 fatty acids** have been studied extensively for about 40 years, by scientists. A year-long study where people took 3 or 4 fish oil capsules a day found a greater improvement in lung capacity than people who didn't take them. But another study showed that high doses of omega-3 supplements could cause a slight decline in lung capacity of some asthmatics. If you try this, use the capsules for at least four weeks. That's the point where good changes start to happen in nearly every study.

Tips on Using Any Medication

Finally, here are a few tips to effectively using any medication. The first is to know the medication you are taking. This includes the side effects, dosage, proper technique for taking it and when to call the doctor if it's not working. Ask your doctor for a photocopy of all of the information on the medicine from the *Physician's Desk Reference*. Ask for an explanation of it. Discuss the drug with your pharmacist, too.

Knowing yourself is a good idea, also. If you can recognize the onset of an allergy or asthma episode and circumvent it, that's ideal. If you are in doubt, contact your physician. It's better to visit the doctor and be told you're all right than to push it and end up in the hospital, or worse.

Medication and your baby

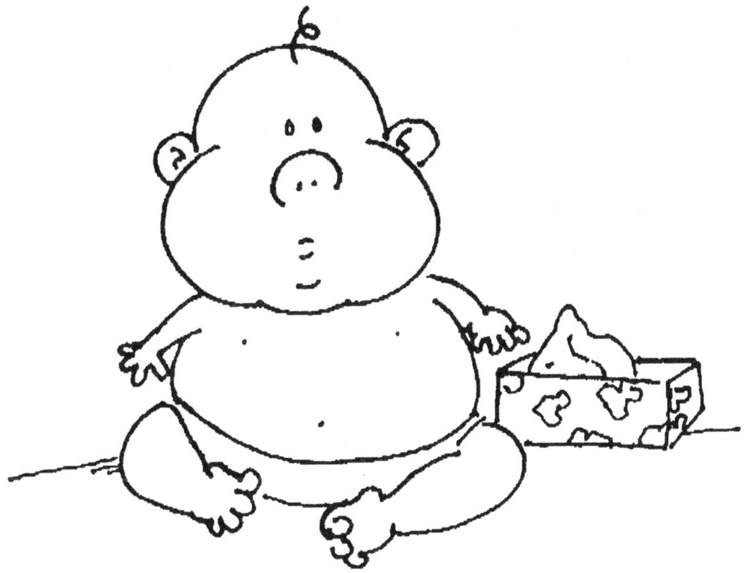

Just how many expectant mothers in the U.S. have asthma? Studies show the number to be between 2% and 4%. Historically, these mothers have been told they're at increased risk for complications including premature delivery, low birth-weight babies, and fetal death. The good news is that with education and management, these moms can have normal, healthy babies. The challenge for the health care providers is finding the ideal treatment program for the individual mother.

Our knowledge of many of the drugs we routinely use is still sketchy. Many physicians are very cautious in their management of asthmatic mothers. The National Asthma Education Program found that "undertreatment of asthma, principally due to unfounded fears of medication, is the major problem in asthma management during pregnancy."

We can't blame our physicians for being overly protective. So, let's look at what medical science *does* know about the drugs we take.

Cromolyn Sodium is an old favorite in asthma prevention. It works by inhibiting the release of histamines and by stabilizing the mast cells. It's believed that less than 10% of this medication enters the mother's bloodstream. There are no studies that report how much of that 10%, if any, can cross the placental membrane to the baby. We do know that many women continue to use their Cromolyn Sodium through out their pregnancy with no apparent ill effects to the baby. It's not the ideal finding, but it's the only one we have to date.

Theophylline is a methylxanthine that relaxes the smooth muscles of the bronchial tree. It seems that the more we learn about this drug, the less we really know about it. Traditionally, we believed that it relaxed the muscles by inhibiting a substance called cyclic AMP. New studies are demonstrating that this isn't so. It was also previously thought that it didn't cross the placental membrane. Recent studies have also proven that to be false. It does cross the membrane, and while there have been no congenital defects, some babies can have a toxic reaction if the blood level concentration is high enough. The reaction can take the form of nausea, vomiting and nervousness.

Theophylline breaks down in the baby's system to a caffeine-like substance which stimulates their respiratory drive. After birth, the baby experiences a withdrawal syndrome that some researchers have suggested is linked to apneic episodes (interruption of breathing) and Sudden Infant Death Syndrome (SIDS). This phenomena is still under investigation. (New research points to a heart defect as another cause of SIDS. Babies sleeping on their bellies is another cause.) The truth is, we just don't know all about it yet.

We also know that the drug not only crosses the placental membrane, but can be passed to the baby via breast milk. While less than 1% of the mother's dosage is transmitted through the milk, it's uncertain what effect this may have on the baby.

Relievers, or **beta agonists** are the most common medications given for the management of asthma. These are usually taken as either an inhaler or an aerosol treatment. The granddaddy of this family of drugs is epinephrine. It's given with caution to expectant mothers. Some physicians may elect to give this medication in instances of asthmatic emergency, or in the event of a severe allergic reaction. It's known to cause an increased heart rate in both the mother and the baby and has been linked to some congenital deformities.

A safer drug, **Albuterol Sulfate**, is a grandchild of epinephrine. This drug is used not only to ease asthma attacks, but also to stop premature labor. Many mothers routinely take it via an inhaler with no reported risk to the baby. We do know that albuterol crosses the placental membrane. Studies have shown no difference in outcome for mothers taking the medication than that of nonasthmatic mothers not taking the drug. The researchers compared the incidences of premature delivery, low birth weight, fetal death, growth retardation, and congenital abnormalities and found no statistical differences. The mothers taking albuterol did have a slight increase in blood pressure, but it didn't seem to affect the fetus.

Part 5
Asthma Management

How to use a peak flow meter to manage your asthma

A peak flow meter is a tool that allows you to keep track of your airway's openness. It's a hand-held device that measures how hard you're able to blow out. By keeping track of this measurement you can keep an eye on how your lungs are doing.

If your peak flow measurement starts to drop out of your normal range it may be a sign that you're about to have an asthma attack. The peak flow meter can't prevent an asthma attack, but, it can signal you to take action before the attack occurs.

Which One Is Right For You?

There are many different types of peak flow meters available. Some are designed to appeal to children, some are more compact and fit into a purse or pocket. All come with instructions. Children as young as five years old successfully use a peak flow meter on a regular basis. Your healthcare provider can and should assist you with the proper way to use yours.

Measurement of peak flow is being incorporated into many asthma management plans. Patients are encouraged to keep a diary and to use their peak flow devices at least twice a day, once in the morning and once in the evening.

If you use an inhaled bronchodilator at home, you should do your measurement before and after taking your treatment in the morning and later in the day. If you're only able to use your peak flow meter once a day, it's recommended that you use it in the morning. By regularly monitoring your measurements, you and your doctor can establish target zones and a management plan.

How to Use Your Peak Flow Meter

A peak flow meter is easy to use. Simply take in a deep breath, place the mouthpiece in your mouth and exhale as hard and as fast as you can. The meter will measure the force with which the air comes out of your lungs. It's measured in Liters per second.

Do the measurement standing up, if possible. This allows the maximum movement of your chest as you blast the air out. If you're seated, or slouching your reading may not be as accurate. Ideally, you'll do three measurements in a row to help you determine your condition at that time. Just doing one often stimulates a cough and may not give you an accurate record of your status.

Know Your Zones

The National Heart, Blood and Lung Institute has developed a zone approach to help patients understand their peak flow measurements and to help standardize care. The zone approach system establishes three colored zones, green, yellow, and red.

You measure your peak flow twice daily for two to three weeks. Your physician or health care provider assists you in determining your ideal peak flow value zone. This is your normal, or green zone. Some daily fluctuation in values is normal, so a range of 80% to 100% of the patients ideal value is determined to be their green zone.

The next range is the yellow zone. You're in this area when your peak flow value is 50% to 80 % of your ideal effort. In this case, you may be beginning to develop an asthmatic reaction. This zone is a signal that some action should be taken to interrupt the asthmatic process and/or prevent it from worsening.

The third zone is a red zone or alert zone. In this case, your peak flow is below 50% of your ideal and immediate action should be taken to respond to your condition.

Step-By-Step Management Plan

Many health care providers will give you a step-by-step plan of management along with the zone monitoring plan, based on your past experiences and responses. For example, if your peak flow is in the upper portion of the yellow zone you should repeat your aerosol therapy. If it improves, return to your regular regimen. If not, then move to the next step, etc.

These tailored programs are proving to be effective management tools. The secret to their success is patient cooperation and the customized design. The danger of these programs is the physician who attempts to force you into a plan that doesn't fit. If your health care provider gives you a plan based solely on a chart or graph and doesn't look at you specifically, find another doctor.

Don't take the plan as gospel. Your plan may work fine most of the time. But, if you hit a time when it doesn't seem to be working, seek medical assistance. No written plan is foolproof, and your health is too important to risk.

There are many factors that influence your ideal peak flow measurement. Height, weight, age, and physical condition are just a few of the considerations that are used to determine your range. Keeping a diary, even after your initial evaluation period, can help you identify subtle and seasonal variations in your asthma. It'll also help your physician regulate your medication.

Peak flow meters are covered by most insurance companies when prescribed by a physician. The cost of the meter is quickly recovered by a decrease in emergency room visits and office visits for patients using the devices. For you, the peak flow meter is an easy, inexpensive tool that can help you monitor and manage your condition and help you head off a serious attack.

My Peak Flow Ranges Are:

GREEN: 80% to 100% of ideal value
Zone ______________________________

YELLOW: 50% to 80% of ideal
Zone ______________________________

RED: Below 50% of ideal **ALERT!**
Zone ______________________________

What You Should Do In Each Peak Flow Zone

(To be completed by your physician)

Green Zone Medication Instructions: ______________________________
____
____
____

Yellow Zone Medication Instructions: ______________________________
____
____
____

Red Zone Medication Instructions: ______________________________
____
____
____

Part 6
Wellness

Pulmonary rehabilitation – a patient's guide

Pulmonary rehab is a way of helping you manage your breathing so you can live an active life. It can't cure your lung condition, but it *can* teach you how to make the most of it. It doesn't mean turning you into an athlete, it does mean helping you be the best you can be.

Many people participate in and benefit from pulmonary rehabilitation programs. Patients with asthma, COPD, bronchitis, bronchiectasis, severe obesity, accident victims, cystic fibrosis patients and some cardiac patients are just a few of the grops of people who have participated in rehab programs. Actors, singers, public speakers, athletes and many people who simply wish to learn about their breathing and make the most of it – all have completed pulmonary rehabilitation programs, too.

> Pulmonary Rehabilitation may be described as an art of medical practice wherein an individually-tailored multidisiplinary program is formulated which through accurate diagnosis, therapy, emotional support, and education, stabilizes or reverses both the physio- and psychopathology of pulmonary disease, and attempts to return the patient to the highest possible functional capacity allowed by his pulmonary handicap and over all life situation."
>
> *American College of Chest Physicians, 1974*

Goals

The scope and content of a successful pulmonary rehabilitation program is as different as each individual participant. The program should be designed for *your* specific needs and address *your* unique situation.

The best way to make the most of your program is to sit down with your practitioner and establish realistic goals for your progress. You should discuss both short-term goals and long-term goals. For example, a good long-term personal goal would be to do your own shopping again. To achieve this, you must be able to drive again, walk up and down the aisles of the store, stand for approximately an hour, and lift grocery objects. So your rehab program should involve building up your stamina and strength, plus learning compensatory breathing skills. These are all sub-goals or short-term goals. Your health care practitioner should be able to help you define these tasks and start you on the road to achieving them.

Your practitioner should also be able to direct you to professionals who are specialists in other areas. If you need adaptive driving equipment or supplemental oxygen, there are specialists who can help you. A big red flag should go up if your practitioner suggests that you don't need assistance from another professional. No one should keep you from seeking a second opinion or additional information from another source.

Multi-Disciplinary Approach

Pulmonary Rehabilitation is more than exercise sessions and a few breathing tricks. It should involve specialists from several disciplines, including, but not limited to respiratory therapy, cardiology, physical therapy, occupational therapy, social services, nutrition, and diabetic specialists. There is no set team makeup. The composition of the team that assists you is determined by your needs. Most programs determine the exact team that a patient needs through a series of interviews and questionnaires. They sit down with you and ask you about your daily activities and needs. It's important that you answer these questions as honestly and completely as possible. Practitioners can't help you fix a problem if they don't know it's a problem. There should be at least one initial interview and frequent follow-up interviews to discuss your progress.

Exercise Sessions

Most rehab programs incorporate exercise sessions. These are usually done two to three times a week and are geared to your current fitness level. The secret to successful exercise sessions is working along with your practitioner.

You'll have good days and bad days – that's normal. It's important that you speak up and let them know when you're having a rough day. It's equally important that you don't overdo it on days that you feel really good. Your practitioner can help you track your progress and help you achieve a steady improvement.

The other secret to getting the most from your exercise sessions is to incorporate home exercise on the days you don't come into the gym. It may only be a series of stretches that your practitioner helps you work out. But it should be a light workout that complements your regular one.

On the very first day you start your exercise program, you should also start your home exercise plan. You should, from the very beginning, be thinking about what you're going to do when you graduate from your rehab program. How are you going to keep in shape and keep up with what you have learned?

The focus of rehab is to help you become the best you can be. If you quit the day you graduate, you're cheating yourself and you really won't have accomplished anything.

Meeting People

Meeting other people with the same problems and illnesses can be very important. No one's going to stand you up and make you discuss intimate details. In most programs, you won't be in a group situation, but you may see other patients with home oxygen or inhalers. Getting to know someone else with the same condition makes you feel less isolated and gives you an opportunity to exchange ideas. It can also help you get through the workout if you have a friend on the same schedule.

Learning New Things

Rehabilitation is your opportunity to ask questions, learn new skills, and get yourself back on your feet. It's done in a safe, controlled medical atmosphere. Believe me, your medical advisors don't want you to have a heart attack while you're exercising. They won't let you do an activity that you're not ready and able to do. You know that disclaimer at the beginning of exercise videos that says you should consult your physician before starting something new? Your doctor referred you to rehab to help you get better, so this is your chance. You'll be taught breathing skills, exercises, and techniques to help you do things. Ask questions, take notes and make the most of it!

Outcomes and Follow-up Visits

Outcomes is the new buzzword in medical circles. Health care service providers now have to prove the services they are providing are successful and beneficial to the patient. This can be very helpful for you.

Insist that your practitioner share with you how you're doing throughout your sessions. Your rehab specialist usually sends regular reports to your physicians, so ask that those reports be discussed with you.

Also insist that you get assistance in developing a maintenance program for when you stop coming to the sessions. There should also be at least one follow-up visit to determine if the rehab program helped you and to see if you are still on track. If one is not scheduled for you, ask for one. As a patient it's your right. You are the consumer and you are their reason for being there. You're entitled to know what the outcome was for your personal rehabilitation program.

Flu vaccines

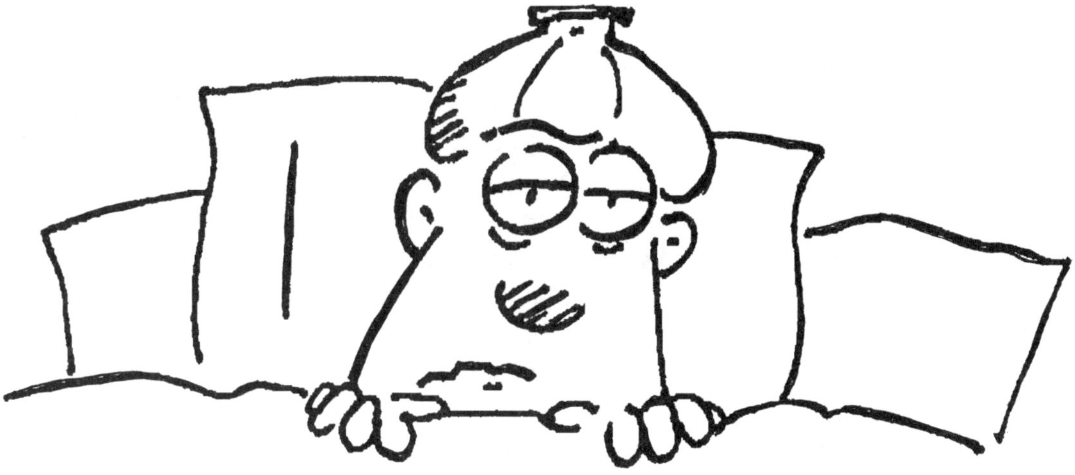

Every fall and winter, flu season comes around. That means it's time for the annual shot that's recommended for most of us. The Centers for Disease Control (CDC) in Atlanta advises anyone over the age of six months, and especially people in high risk groups, be vaccinated. High risk groups include residents of nursing homes or extended care facilities, anyone over the age of 65, health care providers, service industry workers (that wonderful catch-all category that includes anyone who comes in contact with the general public), and family members of individuals in these groups.

The flu is caused not just by a single virus, but by a family of viruses. Every year, the vaccine gets updated with new antigens to cover all the new strains of the flu virus family expected to hit the country. Due to changes in the composition of the vaccine itself, it is stressed that the new version be given. Some health care providers gave the previous years' vaccine until the supply was exhausted, and then switched to the new one. This may be cost effective, but does not guarantee you protection against the illness. Ask your health care provider which version you are getting and insist on the new one!

The new vaccine contains only noninfectious viral agents. It can't cause the flu. It can, however, cause a systemic immune response which may include fever, malaise, and myalgia. Though uncommon, this reaction could begin within six to twelve hours after administration of the vaccine. It may continue up to forty-eight hours. The flu vaccine can be given at the same time as the pneumococcal vaccine.

The recommended time period for administering the vaccine has been extended. In the United States, influenza activity usually peaks between December and early March. It's important to be vaccinated at least one month prior to this time span to insure optimal protection. Vaccination time span now includes the entire month of October and continues through the first two weeks of November. People usually develop an immunity within 30 days and are covered for the entire flu season.

If you have allergic responses to eggs, or previous responses to the flu vaccine, you shouldn't get a flu shot. The vaccine is made using eggs, so allergies to eggs or feathers mean a reaction is possible. (If you've recently had an upper respiratory infection, you'll want to wait before getting vaccinated.)

There are alternatives to the vaccine for the egg-allergic. You can be treated prophylactically with antiviral agents like Amantadine or Rimantadine. These drugs are known to reduce the severity and duration of the flu, if the treatment is begun within 48 hours of the onset of symptoms. The CDC stresses that use of these chemoprophylactics are not without risk of serious side effects. They are not a substitute for vaccination.

Children taking aspirin therapy are particularly susceptible to developing Reye's Syndrome after a case of the flu. There are no specific recommendations for the vaccination of young school age children, and parents are encouraged to discuss vaccination with their pediatrician. Many high schools and colleges are recommending and offering the flu vaccines to their students. There have been no dangers associated with this practice. Businesses provide free flu shots to employees. And many cities have instituted clinics offering free shots for everyone.

Having the flu is miserable. It can also result in more serious medical complications if not closely monitored. When flu season is upon us, get your shot and stay healthy.

Techniques for relaxation and easier breathing

You can use your breathing to improve your overall well-being. It's natural *not* to think about your breathing, but under stress, many of us forget to breathe. This can be a problem for those of us with allergies, and a bigger problem for those of us with asthma. Let's look at the subject, and how paying a little bit of attention to your breathing can pay off.

A Natural Process

Breathing – the simple ebb and flow of air into and out of your body. Most Americans take the process for granted. We breathe, on average, some 28,000 times a day, and we never think about it. In fact, we're so sure our breathing will continue, that we go to bed each night and rarely mention it in our prayers. Yet, breathing is also one of the most studied and perfected physiological functions in the history of humankind.

Breathing has a profound effect on our physical, mental, and spiritual well-being. Take a slow deep breath. It provides fresh oxygen to your body, calms your mind, and, many believe, is a direct link to your soul. In Indian traditions, Yogis have studied and perfected the art of breathing. They call it Pranayama, and writings about the proper practice and technique of breath work date back over 4,000 years. In ancient texts, "Prana" means life-force or energy, and "yama" is to strengthen and lengthen. Breathing is an integral part of the meditative tradition. Ancient wisdom teaches that when breathing is slow, regular, and refined, a state of balance occurs, because Prana is reaching all the levels of our consciousness.

In India, breathing is more than just air moving in and out. "Breath is the junction point of the mind, body, and spirit. Every change of mental state is reflected in the mind and then in the body." Western doctors have made great headway exploring the impact of breathing on the mind-body connection and are advocating advanced breathing techniques for everything from stress reduction to cancer therapy. Among these is Andrew Weil, M.D., author of *Eight Weeks to Optimum Health* and *Spontaneous Healing*. He lists many breathing exercises based on Indian and Chinese traditions. Among these are techniques to rejuvenate, re-energize and relax the body.

Natural breathing is a common term that simply identifies a form of abdominal breathing. It's also sometimes called complete breathing. To correctly perform this type of breathing, lie or sit comfortably with your spine straight. If you are sitting, sit either on the floor or in a chair, and sit forward on the front half of the chair. Do not lean back in the chair, as this will collapse and compress the abdominal muscles and they will not be able to support you as you breathe. If you are lying down, you may want to bend your knees to relieve the pressure from your lower back, and gently tilt the pelvis to push the curve out of your lower spine. Place one hand on your abdomen and the other on your chest. Now slowly breathe in through your nose for a count of ten. As you do so, feel the air gently flow into your body and fill your belly. You should feel the hand on your belly rise as the air flows in. Now hold your breath in for approximately ten seconds. Exhale slowly and completely through your nose. Do not let the air rush out of the body. It should flow out as smoothly as it flowed in. Slowly repeat this breathing technique, and try to keep your attention on the smooth, rhythmic flow of air into and out of your body. It should become cyclic and continuous.

Pursed-lip breathing is another technique you may wish to try. Breathe slowly and deeply in through your nose and out through your mouth. As you exhale, do so through pursed or puckered lips. To get the maximum effectiveness from pursed-lip breathing, you should exhale for twice as long as you inhale. So you may want to modify the count pattern. Try inhaling for four counts and exhaling for eight counts. This breathing exercise is good for both relaxing you and helping you catch your breath during exertion or exercise.

Alternative breathing is another technique that's widely used. To use this skill, sit or lie comfortably as in abdominal breathing. Use the thumb of your right hand to gently push your right nostril closed. Exhale gently through your left nostril and then slowly breathe in through the left nostril. Release your right nostril and close off your left nostril with the forefinger of your right hand. Exhale through the right nostril and then gently inhale. Continue this for ten breaths, alternating nostrils.

Many people, as they get older, have difficulty breathing while doing housework or other basic life tasks. There is a secret to getting things done and keeping your breath about you. It is really very easy, but also easy to forget. Here it is: breathe on the exertion. If you're preparing to move a heavy box or do any type of physical activity, take a deep breath and begin the activity as you exhale. Think of it as stocking up your store of oxygen and then starting. The other thing many people forget to do is to continue breathing. They lift something heavy and they hold their breath while they do it. One secret that combines these two skills is to begin pursed lip breathing with a steady rhythm and continue it throughout the exertion. In other words, breathe in 2,3,4; breathe out, 2,3,4; breathe in 2,3,4; Lift, breathe out 2,3,4; breathe in 2,3,4; etc. It sounds silly, but sometimes we really do forget to breathe, and it makes the physical work we do harder, causing us to lose our breath.

Visualization Techniques

Combining deep breathing techniques with visualization is gaining popularity in the West. Guided imagery tapes and books can be found in most book and audio stores. Video tapes with meditation and imagery techniques can be purchased or rented from most stores. Tapes incorporating basic yoga stretches and breathing include Dixie Carter's *Unworkout* and several by film star Raquel Welch. Shirley MacLaine's tape and book, *Going Within*, explores the Eastern concept of "chakras" or life energy centers. This program has breathing/meditation exercises that use the visualization of breathing in colors to different parts of the body. Chakras are the seven energy centers inside your body. They correspond to the seven life centers and to the seven colors of the rainbow. By breathing in colors and energy to these centers, you can then release their energy and promote overall health, healing and well being.

Breathing is an integral component of our lives. If you don't believe that, just try stopping for a few minutes and see how long you last. Many breathing techniques find their roots in Eastern traditions. Sages and yogis say they have reached heightened states through the employment of various breathing skills. Whether you're looking for heightened awareness or just a way to sanely get through your e-mail, you can learn from their techniques. Ideally, the skills should be practiced every day. In many Eastern traditions, they're only a part of a lifestyle that many Westerners would find difficult to adopt. The traditions encompass diet standards, exercise and meditative practices. The secret is to find the best options for you and to stick to them. Select the practices that work in your life and incorporate them into your daily routine. Remember, if you miss a day, that's okay. The Eastern traditions teach, above all, balance and moderation as their objectives – two aspects of life so many of us in the West are in search of.

Avoiding illness

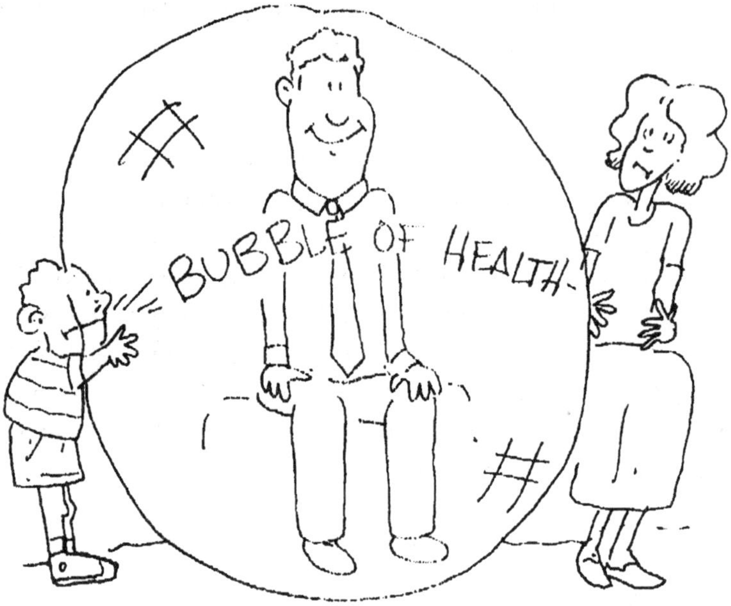

Now you know how your immune system works, but how do you know when your immune system is working? Unfortunately, you won't know your immune system isn't working until it's challenged by an illness. And living through the immune response isn't all that fun anyway.

In my mind, it's easier to prevent challenges to the immune system than to let the immune response run its course of producing different antibodies, inflammation, congestion, etc.

Living sensibly, eating right, exercising regularly and sleeping will help keep your body in a state of good health, and that helps keep illness away.

But the truth is, our lives today don't always permit this to happen. And if it's a child with asthma we're talking about, forget it. The kid is going to want to do what his friends do. The key to keeping children healthy is knowing when they're getting sick and how to stop the illness before it becomes a major crisis.

Keeping Your Lungs Healthy

The first step is to keep your lungs in a clean environment. Avoid smoky rooms, don't breathe chemical fumes or pollutants, and give up smoking if you haven't already. A HEPA air filter can help keep the air you breathe pure and clean.

Step two is to avoid unhealthy people. Sometimes they can't be avoided, but if your friend has the flu or a cold, keep a good distance away. Many viruses and bacteria are spread by droplets. When the infected person coughs or sneezes, ask him to cover his mouth and nose. Avoid shaking hands and be sure to wash your hands well after contact and especially before eating.

Get Your Shots

An annual flu shot and a pneumonia shot (good for 10 years) can boost your immunity against these common diseases. Flu vaccines are specifically formulated for the two or three strains of flu that scientists think are most likely to infect the U.S. in the coming season. That's why you have to be vaccinated annually – for continued protection against newer strains. It's also a good idea to remember to take the shot early in the flu season. It takes about 30 days to build up an immunity to the flu. If you wait until someone at your office or school has the flu before you get the shot, it's too late.

Keep Coughing And Deep Breathing

If you feel you're coming down with something, keep coughing and deep-breathing. The lungs are an ideal place for a bug to set up housekeeping. The neighborhood is moist, dark and quiet, unless you shake things up by periodically taking deep breaths and opening up your airways. Coughing keeps the lungs clean and clear of debris and doesn't give the infection much of an opportunity to establish itself.

Adjust Your Exercise – And Take Care of Yourself!

If you have a regular exercise routine you may wish to modify it slightly. Continuing to exercise is important, but sometimes, giving your body time to rest and recover is a good idea, too. (Your physician might have some good advice on that, as well.)

Eat right, drink plenty of fluids, and get some rest. That's good advice any time, but more so if your immune system is trying to fight off an invader. Lay off burning the candle at both ends and stop eating junk foods. Be a little more aware of your diet and help your body restore itself. And don't forget the comfort food. Chicken soup really does have something in it that helps speed up the immune response.

It's trite but true: laughter is the best medicine. It relieves stress and gives your lungs a good workout. Rent a movie, watch an old sitcom, read a funny book or call a friend who makes you laugh.

Crying is not a bad idea either. It relieves stress and most people take nice deep breaths when they cry. But it can also stuff up your nose.

Then there's the old Korean remedy for respiratory illness: spicy food. When you feel your body under attack, eat spicy food and blow your nose a lot. The Jewish alternative, as suggested by a friend's Great-Aunt Anna: buy some snuff (chewing tobacco) and snort a pinch. It'll make you sneeze out everything. (Hey, it worked for her, and she lived to be 94!)

Don't Stop Your Medications

Continue your prescribed medications. A mistake many asthma and allergy sufferers make is to discontinue their medications when they feel well – or they're not as vigilant and miss a few days. This sets them up for an infection. Allergy sufferers, in particular, feel they can stop their medication when pollen season is past. If this is your plan, discuss it with your allergist. For safety reasons, you may want to taper off your medication rather than stop cold turkey. Each allergy and asthma sufferer is unique and requires a tailored program for starting or stopping medication.

Listen To Your Body

How do you know if you're getting an infection? Listen to your body and it'll tell you. Some common signs include feeling tired or run down, restlessness or irritability, a sore throat or cough, difficulty breathing or a tightness in the chest, fever or chills, achiness, weight loss or gain, swelling of your ankles or legs, an increased heart rate at rest, and a feeling of doom or persistent feelings that you are not quite right. In addition, since you're probably quite sinus-aware, you'll see a change in the color or consistency of your sinus drainage or sputum. Clear or white is okay, any other color means trouble. Also watch for wheezing or shortness of breath.

If you experience any of these symptoms, call your doctor right away. Continue to take your regular medications unless the doctor instructs you otherwise. Make sure your doctor and pharmacist are aware of the medications you're on now, and ask about conflicts with anything else your doctor wants to prescribe.

Above all, listen to your body. It knows when something's amiss.

Coping with life when breathing is tough

Working smarter is almost a commandment in the business world. A lot of the skills that we use in the office are really common sense, when you think about them. If you're a pulmonary patient, you need some extra help. Working smarter around the house and in other activities can give you that extra oomph you need to make it through the day. Working smarter boils down to three basics: conserve your energy, pace yourself, and use your skills to their fullest potential.

Energy Conservation

Conserving energy is really eliminating the unnecessary steps, or combining repetitive steps in a procedure. For example, if you're going to make a salad, get the lettuce, tomatoes, and cucumbers out of the refrigerator and take them to the sink for washing all at the same time. Then move them all to the table and sit down and chop them one after the other. This is much more efficient than getting the lettuce out of the refrigerator, washing and chopping it, then going back for the tomatoes, washing and chopping them ...

Folding clothes can also be simplified. Don't wash a load of whites, fold them, put them away and go back to do the colors. Wash a load, put it on your bed and go about your business. Later, when all the clothes have been washed and are ready for folding, you can sit on the bed and do them all at once. This is much more efficient than spending an entire day getting up and walking all over the house putting things away.

The rules of thumb for energy conservation are: assemble all your tools/supplies first; cut down on the repetitive jobs (walking back and forth) as much as possible; sit whenever possible; and pace yourself.

Pacing Yourself

Pacing yourself is important. Take your time! Even race car drivers know that, for the long haul, they sometimes need to sit back and wait. So do you! When you hurry, you frequently don't take deep breaths, and you become flustered. Then you become short of breath. Pace yourself, take your time and schedule breaks for resting. This is just as important in the little activities as in the big ones.

If housework tires you out, plan on doing one room at a time. Vacuum the living room, take a breather (literally) and then start the bedroom. Or vacuum today and dust tomorrow.

If you know going to the grocery store is tiring for you, particularly in the summer heat, plan to go in the early morning before the heat gets bad. Also, plan to come home and take a short break before you unload the groceries. Take fifteen minutes immediately upon returning home to sit down and rest for a minute. Your groceries can wait, and they'll be fine. If you're concerned about ice cream melting or milk spoiling, just ask the cashier to put them in separate bags then bring those in with you, but let the rest wait a few minutes.

Using Your Skills to Your Best Advantage

This really is easier than it sounds. Basically, it means applying all that you have learned about your breathing to your daily activities. It means thinking about your activities before you do them, and figuring out the best way for you to get them done. Forget about the way you would have done it when you were twenty. You have to deal with things the best way you can right now. So don't overextend yourself and don't forget to breathe. One of the biggest secrets is to remember to take a nice, slow breath in and exhale on the exertion. No matter what you're doing – if it's reaching, wiping, or lifting, take slow breaths and do the work on the exhale.

Lifting

Have you ever noticed how, sometimes when you pick things up, you hold your breath? The smart way to pick something up is to take a few, deep breaths through pursed lips – take a big breath in and exhale through pursed lips as you pick up the object. Remember to take another breath in. It's easiest to breathe in a counted rhythm. For example, breathe in: 1,2,3; breathe out: 1,2,3,4,5,6; breathe in: 1,2,3; lift and breathe out: 1,2,3,4,5,6: breathe in: 1,2,3, etc. Remember to breathe out for twice as long as you breathe in.

Drying Dishes

Don't do it! There's no reason to. They can dry in a rack. You don't have to do all the unnecessary work of rubbing each and every one with a towel. If you have a dishwasher, use it! They save energy in the long run.

Cooking

There are many microwave and simplified cookbooks available. Many of your old favorite dishes can be prepared in easier, less time-consuming ways. Single-pot cooking and slow cookers can also be a godsend. Use them! If you must cook something on top of the stove that requires tending, use a stool or chair and sit down in between stirring.

Give yourself a break. We've already discussed the proper way to cut vegetables. In some instances, you can also use frozen vegetables that don't need cutting or peeling. Also, frozen dinners have come a long way. You can now buy frozen vegetable casseroles and other dishes that don't require a great deal of preparation other than warming in the oven.

Bathing

The heat and humidity changes involved in bathing can be rough. If possible, add handrails or a stool to your bathtub. When you finish your bath or shower, before hopping out of the tub, stop for a minute and take a few deep breaths. Give your body the opportunity to adjust to the temperature changes before you ask it to spring into action. Then climb out of the tub and sit down. I cannot stress enough how important this is.

The bathroom is a very easy place to slip and fall no matter what age you are. It's also a very unforgiving place to fall. Bathrooms are usually close quarters, filled with unforgiving porcelain structures. In *Don Quixote*, there's a line that says, "Whether the stone hits the pitcher or the pitcher hits the stone, it is going to be bad for the pitcher." That's kind of what the bathroom's like. The last thing you want to do is fall and hurt yourself. If you did, you'd likely need medical attention in a hurry, you may not have a phone handy, and you'd probably still be in all your naked glory. So, don't risk it!

The actual process of bathing can be simplified by using a bath mitt. Using a bar of soap to lather yourself up, then a following with a wash cloth involves extra steps. You can purchase a mitt, or you can make one by stitching two wash cloths together on three sides, then soap up the mitt and rub it over you.

Some people find working with a bar of soap difficult. They drop it and then have to bend over to pick it up. One idea to help with this is to switch to liquid soap. Another is to add a suction cupped hook to the shower and use soap on a rope. One inventive woman I know combined all of these ideas. She took two washcloths and sewed them together with a flap, kind of like a sandwich bag. Then she put the soap inside and put a cord on it. She looped the cord to the towel rack in the back of her shower. This may be a little elaborate for you, but the important thing is that it worked for her and she took the time to figure out exactly what she needed.

Drying yourself can also be strenuous work, but it doesn't have to be. Go out today and buy yourself a luxurious terry cloth robe. When you finish bathing, don't dry yourself, just put on the robe and let it do the work. It's made of the same material as a towel, so it works the same way. Climb out of the tub, put your robe on, and sit down for a few minutes. You may still have to dry your toes, but this, too, will be less strenuous since you're already sitting. When you're done, turn the robe inside out and hang it to dry, just as you would a towel.

You may complain that there's no place to sit in the bathroom and no place for a stool. Well, the toilet lid is good for more than keeping the dog from drinking. Put the lid down and have a seat.

Dressing

Getting dressed can be a challenge. An easy way to help yourself through this is to assemble all the clothes you're going to wear – shoes, socks, shirt, pants, undies, etc. Lay them out on the bed, then sit down and begin to put them on. Remember to take regular pursed-lip breaths and to take your time. Refrain from wearing tight, constricting clothes. Shoes that slip on are usually easier than those that tie. It's also a good idea to stay away from leather-soled shoes. They're easy to slip and fall in on wet or slick floors.

Eating

It's one of life's greatest pleasures. It's something to be enjoyed. If you find that you get short of breath or that you have difficulty, perhaps you're eating too fast. One technique is to take a pursed lip breath, inhale again, pause, and then place the food in your mouth. Chew it well and swallow. Then exhale. Doing it this way gives you the opportunity to get a good breath and get some more air in before you place food in your mouth.

Chewing, swallowing, and then exhaling also protects your airway a little. You don't want to try to swallow and inhale at the same time. That increases the likelihood that the food could go down the wrong pipe and choke you.

Another adaptation of this technique is to place the food in your mouth and tuck your chin down on your neck as you chew and swallow. This also helps protect the airway.

If you have difficulty with choking on food, be sure to sweep your mouth out with your tongue. To do this, simply run your tongue along the inside and outside of your teeth. The goal is to dislodge any small food particles that may have become stuck. By cleaning your mouth out, you decrease the likelihood that they will come loose later and go down the wrong way.

Speaking

Talking can sometimes make you very short of breath, especially when you get excited. But speaking and breathing is really easy. In fact, you've already learned the secret, you just may not realize it. Remember that 1:2 ratio you learned when you read about pursed-lip breaths? When you speak, you can speak for the second half of that ratio comfortably. For example, breathe in for a count of three and out for a count of six, then try taking in a deep breath for three and speaking for a count of six. It will take practice, and some getting used to but, but soon you'll be speaking away with no problems. Your family won't be able to get a word in edge-wise!

Stairs

Whether you have stairs in and around your home or not, you need to know how to negotiate them, if only for safety's sake. If you went to your doctor's office and the building caught on fire, how would you get out? You could do it!

While going up the stairs, take in a deep pursed-lip breath and exhale as you step up. Stop when your exhalation runs out. Take in a deep breath and step up again. You may only be able to do one or two stairs at a time, but the important thing is that you pace yourself and coordinate your breathing. You go down the stairs the same way. The key here is to breathe on the exertion, collect yourself, take a deep breath and do it again.

Bending

This is a tough one, but it's not impossible. Again it's just a matter of coordinating your body movement with your breathing. Take a deep, pursed-lip breath in and bend as you exhale. Once down there, you may need to stop for a minute and let your body adjust to the new position. You should take as deep a breath as possible while you're bent over, too. Don't hold your breath. Just take your time and breathe through the movement, remembering to exhale on the exertion.

Reaching Overhead

This can be tricky. Your natural instincts may get in the way of your anatomy. When you look up, you raise your chin, which pulls the front of the larynx up – and pulls your vocal cords tight. The vocal cords pull across your airway and actually block it to some degree.

The way to solve this problem is to look up, get a good idea of what you're reaching for, then tuck your chin down, take a pursed-lip breath in, and reach up as you exhale. The even smarter way is to use a small stool, so you don't have to reach up at all.

Posture

Finally, let me say a few words about the benefits of good posture. Sitting up straight can help your breathing immeasurably. It allows your body to utilize the primary muscles of breath in the most efficient manner. If you slump, or hunch over, it makes it harder for you to breathe. So sit up straight, hold your head up, and breathe easier!

Breathing easy ... during the winter holidays

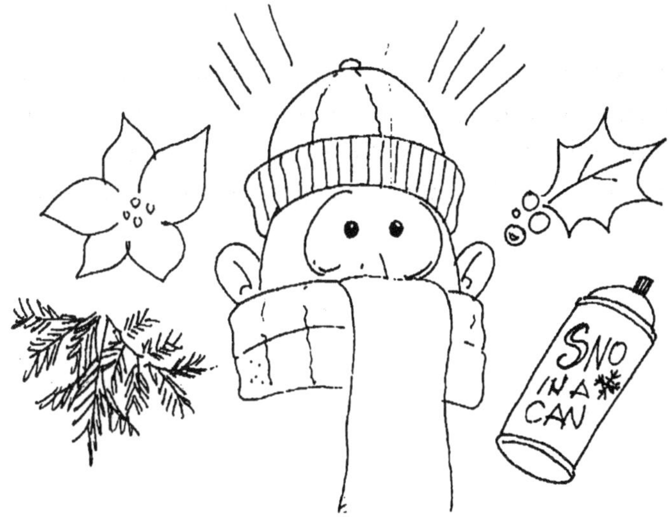

All too soon, the Christmas season will be upon us. The holidays are a time to gather family and friends, one and all, and celebrate with beloved traditions. Allergy and asthma sufferers, however, often find the time-honored traditions must be endured rather than enjoyed. It doesn't have to be that way, though. Here are some helpful hints to get you through the seasonal sniffles.

Beware of Cold Air

Beware of cold, dry air. It's often irritating to the airway and can trigger an asthma attack, making you anything but jolly. When venturing outdoors, bundle up and stay warm. Don't deprive your child (or yourself) of the glory of making snow angels. Just keep an eye on your little one, and don't let him overdo. Watch for signs of overexertion and fatigue. Make sure everyone drinks plenty of fluids and keeps hydrated.

It's a good idea to wrap a muffler or scarf over your nose and mouth to warm the air and keep moisture in. Take care to select a 100% cotton or synthetic fiber fabric if you're allergic to wool. Even wool blends can be irritating when worn as a filter over the nose.

Watch Your Peak Flows

Keeping tabs on your peak flows if you are an asthma sufferer is a good idea. Preventing an asthma attack before it happens is the best medicine. We all love to cuddle up in front of a warm, cozy, cracklin' fire. A wood-burning fire, though, can be just as aggravating to allergy sufferers as cigarette smoke. Gas logs are a good alternative for some, but they too have their hazards. Researchers have documented fumes and emissions from gas logs that can be irritating to some discerning noses.

Holiday room fresheners, simmering pots and potpourri can also be trouble. The propellants found in some room fresheners can be irritating and act as a trigger to a serious reaction. It's best to avoid these if you are sensitive.

Shopping, Wrapping And Decorating

Shopping can also be hazardous if you encounter that evil woman who sprays perfume on everyone within a ten foot radius. Stay away from her, even if you don't have allergies! It's hard to say what's in that spray, and you won't find out you're allergic until it's too late and you've already been exposed.

Did you know that some wrapping paper and tape can cause allergic responses? So can licking the envelopes on your cards. During the year, the average individual may seal one or two envelopes at a time. But the high number of Christmas cards dramatically increases their exposure to the glue. In some rare cases envelope glue has caused extreme anaphylactic reactions requiring emergency medical assistance. Most people only experience a thick feeling in their tongue or a rash from handling the tape. But why take the chance? There are great new glue sticks out specifically for sealing envelopes. Check your local office supply store.

Care should be used when decorating. From the allergist's perspective, holiday greenery often causes an allergic reaction if not handled properly. Poinsettias are poisonous. They not only can cause a rash from touching them, but can be fatal if ingested. Ivy, holly and chrysanthemums also can cause these types of reactions. So please, wear gloves if trimming or arranging the greens. Latex allergy sufferers, take care with the gloves you select.

The Christmas tree itself, the very symbol of the Yule season, can also be a source of allergens. Tree allergies are very common. Many sufferers may be allergic to pines, but tolerate firs very well. If you've ever been tested for allergies, generic tree testing was probably part of the regimen. Call your doctor and ask for the result of your tests before you bring home a tree you can't live with.

THOU SHALT NOT FLOCK! If there is an allergy sufferer in your home, avoiding flocked trees is a good idea. It's often hard to identify the chemicals used in the professionally-flocked trees and the do-it-yourself versions usually have propellants to make the flock stuff spray. Both varieties can be irritating.

Artificial trees are a good alternative, providing they have been stored properly. When not carefully packed, artificial trees often collect dust and become an ideal host for dust mites. One approach to making your tree allergy-free is to set it up on the patio and let it air out before bringing it into the house. When you pack the tree up after Christmas, wrap each part in plastic garbage bags to protect them from dust and make next year's airing easier.

Eating And Drinking

Eating is an integral part of holiday festivities. There are many alternatives to traditional Christmas fare for those who are sensitive or have diet restrictions. People suffering from food allergies are caught in a dead heat over eggnog. About 50% are allergic to the egg and about 50% are allergic to the nog (milk and dairy products). The nutmeg seems to be safe, though.

Wassail, an apple cider alternative, is good for most people. Just be aware that many recipes we looked at call for nutmeg, ginger, mace, cloves, allspice, cinnamon, egg whites and egg yolks, brandy and sherry – all potential allergens.

Other foods that may worry allergy sufferers are citrus fruits, coconut, bananas, figs, shellfish, and celery. At last, you have a good excuse to not eat that fruitcake! And watch out, you nut-allergic readers. Nuts seem to be in just about every recipe at holiday-time. Did you know that cranberries can cause a rash from handling them?

Even the holiday turkey should be a prime suspect in some households. Some self-basting varieties may contain chemicals and preservatives which can trigger severe allergic reactions and asthma attacks. Peanut oil is a major culprit of these responses. So read your labels carefully and watch the birdie. (Even better, try one of the free-range, natural, no-preservative turkeys.)

Imbibing at holiday parties is almost a tradition in and of itself. Alcohol can dehydrate, though, and increase the likelihood of an asthma attack. Even in moderation, drinking can be a problem. Often we are unaware until it's too late.

We all know that wines can contain sulfites that may trigger headaches and allergic responses. So those who know this from painful experience usually abstain. But many holiday dishes can be prepared with the wine (see wassail, above), so take care when selecting nibbles. If you do plan to partake, prepare yourself. Drink plenty of non-alcoholic fluids and eat something first.

There's some good news for those of us who still believe in Santa Claus. U.S. astronauts spent over 6 hours attaching dust collectors to the Russian space station MIR. Though the final draft of their study is pending, the preliminary word is that dust and cosmic grit do not pose an allergy threat. So Santa is safe, at least while he's in the air! (Don't ask about chimney soot.)

Perhaps the best advice for the holidays is, don't overdo and take care of yourself.

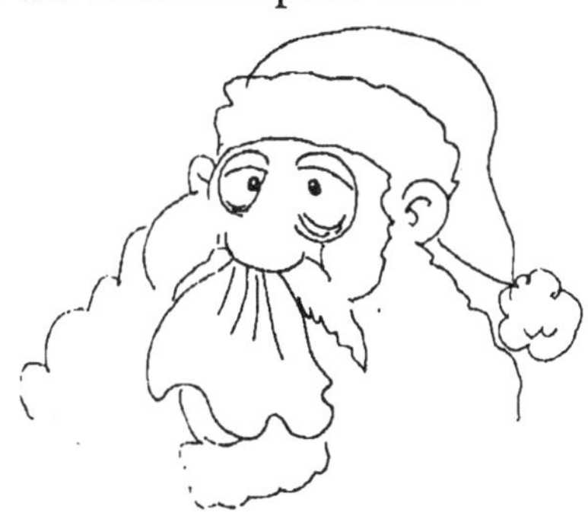

Travel tips

Traveling is one of life's pleasures. It's also one of the dreams that we all plan to fulfill as we grow older. Having a breathing problem doesn't mean you have to forfeit that dream, it just means you have to plan a little more.

Medications are important to take along on your trip. You don't want to be in a strange city and run out of your medication. Finding a physician and a pharmacy in a strange city are a hassle. Refill your medications prior to your departure and bring a copy of your prescriptions with you.

There are many medication nebulizers that are designed for individuals on the go. Some are battery-powered and some can be plugged into your car's cigarette lighter. If you intend to fly and will need to take a nebulizer treatment, the airline can usually make provisions to assist you. It's a good idea to carry MDI versions of your nebulized medication as a back-up supply.

Bring along a **Medication Plan** (see Appendix) that explains what medication you take, the amount, frequency, and reasons why you take it. The paper should also include an emergency contact and your physician's name and telephone number. This is a safety precaution. If you were involved in an accident and couldn't speak for yourself, this paper could assist emergency personnel in treating you. It's an especially good idea if you have asthmatic children.

Oxygen patients can also successfully travel with a little pre-planning. Whether you use a refillable liquid oxygen system or cylinders, you *can* travel. The first step in planning your trip is to speak to your home oxygen supply company. Many companies have reciprocal agreements and networks with companies in other states. They'll assist you and provide you with refills at your destination.

If you're traveling by car or recreational vehicle, ask about systems designed for use in motor vehicles. If you're planning a cruise, speak to the cruise line when you book your trip. Most permit you to bring your own oxygen equipment along.

Airlines are also very accommodating, and will work with you in planning your trip. It's important that you let them know precisely what your needs are and if you are planning to bring additional equipment. There are regulations about how some equipment must be transported and the airline must know in advance so they can provide for your needs. It is also a good idea to allow yourself a little extra time before your flight departure. Your equipment may have to undergo a safety inspection and you don't want this to make you miss your flight!

Food and Drink

Traveling is fun and exciting, but it's also a change in your daily routine. Try to eat and drink just as you would at home. This doesn't mean that you can't try local cuisine, but try to keep yourself on a regular schedule, and remember to drink plenty of fluids. Airlines will provide meals to suit special diets if you request them in advance.

Pace Yourself

Take your time and enjoy your travels. Don't try to cover too much ground at once and don't overdo. Get plenty of rest and avoid stressing yourself out too much.

Maintain Your Routine

If you're a regular exerciser, don't skip those workouts. They'll keep you on track and feeling good. Besides, if you stop your exercises for two or three weeks, it'll be harder to restart when you get home.

Check Your Insurance

Before traveling, it's a good idea to check with your health insurance company to verify that you have coverage at your destination. You don't want to find yourself hospitalized and then having to pay the bill to boot. Office visits and emergency room services can add up quickly. Many companies have short-term travel riders that can be added to a policy if you travel outside your coverage area.

Bring Advanced Directives

If you or a traveling companion has made a decision that you do not wish to be kept alive by extraordinary means, bring a copy of this paperwork (Living Will) with you. Also, discuss it with your travel companions. They don't have to know all the details, just that you have a sealed envelope with you that contain your wishes should you become involved in an accident or become ill.

Going Out of the Country?

International travel isn't out of the question, either. Prior to leaving however, you should do all of the precautions above and a few more. You should investigate the medical conditions in the country to which you will be traveling. A good way to start is by contacting the country's embassy here in the U.S. and ask for information about their services. You should also contact the traveler's assistance division of the U.S. State Department for any travel advisories to that country. And finally, give your insurance company a call to coordinate care prior to departure. Don't assume that your policy has provisions for foreign care, or for flying you home on a medical emergency plane (although there are insurance policies you can get for that).

Exercisers and airway clearance devices

Keeping your airways clean is essential to overall good health. The problem for most patients with pulmonary illness is that mucus collects and clogs up the airway. It prevents air from going in and out and needed oxygen from getting into the body, makes breathing harder, and provides the perfect environment for germs to set up housekeeping and cause an infection. One of the secrets to keeping your airways open and clear is taking care of yourself. Regular exercise requires you to take deep breaths and opens the airways. Eating right and getting plenty of fluids is another secret. Exercising your lungs by taking deep breaths is another way to keep your airways open. Here are some techniques you can practice.

Cough!

Coughing is nature's way of helping you keep your airway clean. When you cough your diaphragm contracts and pushes upward suddenly. This creates a blast of air through your airway, which pushes foreign objects and mucus out. Coughing is a normal response to something going down the wrong way, or to something irritating your airway.

Practicing your cough, and doing it on a regular basis, really can help you keep your lungs in good shape. Believe it or not, there's a right way and a wrong way to cough. When you're trying to cough, always take a deep breath and fully expand your lungs. A cough that comes from the throat is ineffective and will cause you to strain your vocal cords. It may also give you a sore throat.

A good coughing exercise is to sit or stand straight, and place your hands on your tummy. Take three pursed-lip breaths. Exhale completely on the third breath, and take a deep, slow breath in through your nose. Lean forward slightly, pushing in on your abdomen. Cough. Relax, take three pursed-lip breaths, and repeat if needed.

The second exercise to help improve your coughing skills is the Puff Cough. Sit or stand up straight and take in three slow purse-lipped breaths. Exhale completely. Take a slow, deep inhalation through your nose. As you exhale, say the word Puff forcefully. Many books describe this exercise using the word Huff instead of Puff. That's okay, but the P sound is usually a little gentler on the vocal cords and less likely to give you a sore throat. Either word will work, though. This technique is often combined with deep breathing and called the Forced Exhalation Technique, or Active Cycle of Breathing.

Incentive Spirometry

There are many different types of Incentive Spirometers available. Basically, they're all the same. They are tubelike plastic gadgets with a disk or ball inside. As you breathe in, the ball or disk moves up to measure the amount of air you inhaled. These devices provide little or no resistance to your breathing. They're good ways to exercise your lungs by taking a deep breath. They're also a good way to get a rough estimate of your lung volume. In other words, if you normally take ten to fifteen breaths on your spirometer at a volume of 2000 cc each, and you suddenly are only able to take ten breaths at a volume of 700 cc or less, than it's probably a sign that something is going on inside your lungs.

If you decide on a spirometer as your exerciser, you should use it at least two or three times a day. Try to take ten breaths at a time. More is better, providing the breaths are consistent, deep and controlled. The *quality* of the breaths you take is much more important than the quantity.

Positive Expiratory Pressure

Positive Expiratory Pressure is a nice way of exhaling against a pressure. The benefit of this is that it holds your airway open and allow the mucus to unstick itself. Pursed-lip breathing also does this, but using a device that creates resistance is a little more effective. The PEP device usually has a spring and a diaphragm in it. The spring is adjustable and allow you to alter the tension of the resistance, so you can make it harder or easier to blow out against.

PEP devices can be used as exercisers as well as to assist in coughing. To use the PEP as an exerciser, first take ten pursed-lip breaths as a warm-up, then take ten PEP breaths, ten coughs, and ten more pursed-lip breaths. You may rest at any time during this sequence. Pursed-lip breaths will help you catch your breath if you begin to feel short of breath.

Inspiratory Muscle Trainers

Inspiratory Muscle Trainers, or IMT's, are very similar to PEP devices. Basically, they're constructed the same way, but they're used in just the opposite manner. Instead of breathing out against the resistance, you breath in against the resistance. The device has a spring inside and allows you to make the resistance higher, thus making it harder to breathe in against. The idea is that the harder it gets to breathe in, the more exercise your pulmonary muscles get.

It's a good idea to use your IMT every day. One good sequence of exercise is to begin by taking ten pursed-lip breaths, ten IMT breaths, and then ten pursed-lip breaths. This sequence can be done two or three times a day, or as you feel you need it. Adjust your IMT to a higher level as it becomes easier. Just be sure you don't move too quickly. Once you adjust your IMT, it's a good idea to work at that level for at least a week before you move up to the next level. The idea is to condition your lungs gradually and build up your lung strength.

Flutter Device

Up until now, the devices and gadgets we've been discussing have primarily been exercisers that have the secondary effect of helping you cough. The Flutter® device, however, is purely a cough-inducer. It was developed to help cystic fibrosis patients move the thick secretions out of their lungs. The Flutter has been successfully used by other pulmonary patients, too.

The design is a very simple one. Essentially, it's a pipe with a ball inside. When you breathe out, the ball moves up and causes a rattling or fluttering. This fluttering is transmitted into your airway and shakes the secretions loose. The shaking is kind of like when you are mixing up a cake to bake and you tap the spoon, full of batter, on the side of the bowl to shake off the excess. The Flutter uses the same idea, only it's mucus inside of your lungs that you're shaking loose.

Vibration and Chest Physical Therapy

Vibration does from the outside what the Flutter device does from the inside. It shakes the chest wall and causes the secretions to break loose so you can cough them up.

Some of you may associate this technique with cupping or clapping the chest. Actually, cupping and vibration are two different techniques, but they have the same purpose: breaking the mucus loose. Those techniques are more commonly known as Chest Physical Therapy, or CPT. Basically, you cup your hand into a bowl-like shape and strike the patient on the ribs firmly, in a rhythmic pattern. There are some hazards associated with cupping, including breaking a rib or causing damage to the heart and lungs. Before you try this technique, get some instruction from a respiratory care professional.Then you'll know the right places to cup, and the right way to do it. Done incorrectly, you can cause permanent, serious damage.

In more recent years, mechanical and electronic vibrators have been used to provide the same movement of the chest wall. These are special devices developed for medical usage. A good athletic massager can be used in the home setting with the same results. Again, for safety's sake, ask your healthcare provider for training before you try this on your own.

Postural Drainage

Postural Drainage takes advantage of gravity to help you get the mucus out. You simply position yourself in such a way that the different areas of your lungs "drain." The mucus flows into the main airway and toward your mouth, so you can cough it up more easily. It's an old standby, and often used with chest physical therapy. The positions are shown below, and if you're going to use them, remember to take nice, deep pursed-lip breaths and use the coughing techniques while in these positions. Some of these positions may cause discomfort if you have back problem or arthritis. If the position is uncomfortable, don't do it. There are other ways to keep your lungs clean.

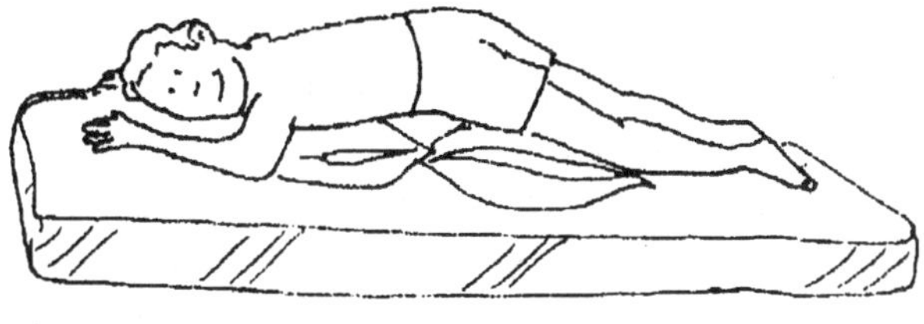

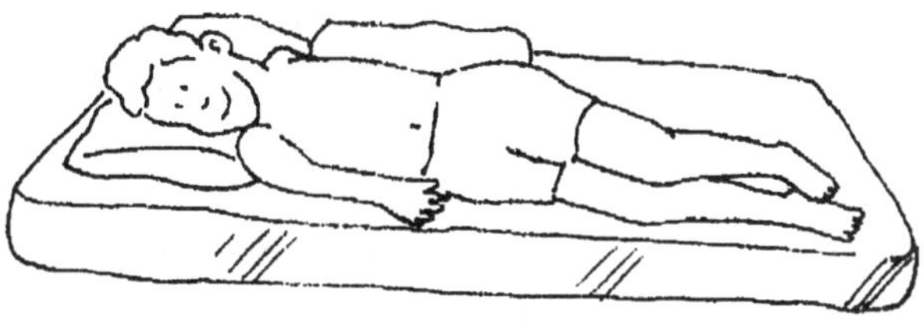

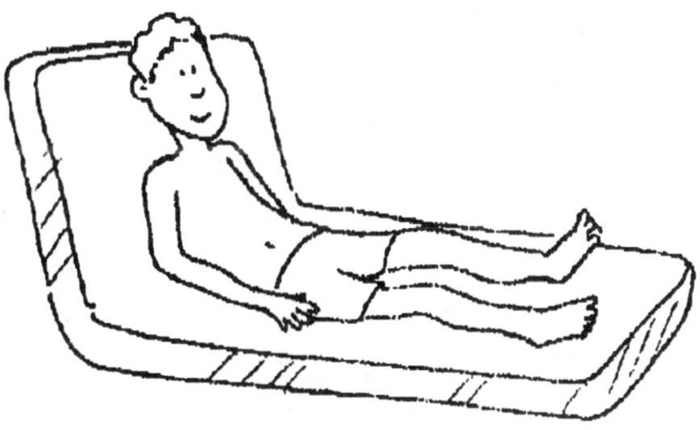

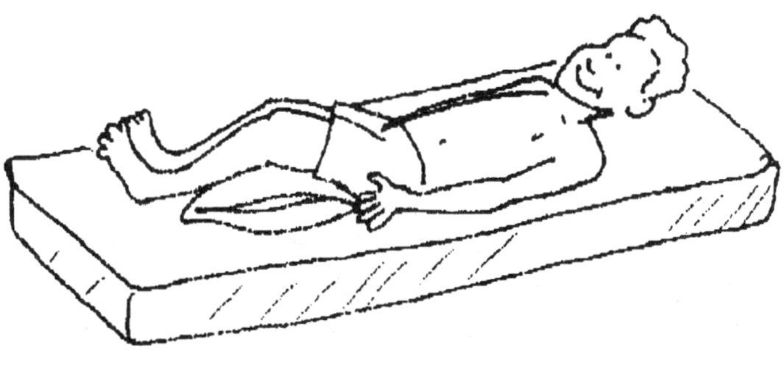

Part 7
Appendices

Your Peak Flow Graph

Name________ Baseline or Personal Best Reading________

Green Zone = Best x 0.8 or above = ________ Yellow Zone = Best x 0.5 or above = ________ Red Zone = Best x 0.5 or below

RECORD YOUR PEAK FLOW TWICE A DAY ON THIS GRAPH

DATE

750 700 650 600 550 500 450 400 350 300 250 200 150 100 50

Your travel medical chart

Name ____
Address ____
City/State/Zip ____
Social Security Number ____
In Case of Emergency, Contact ____
Emergency Phone ____
Physician ____
Physician's Phone ____
Allergies ____
____
Diagnosis ____
____
Insurance Company/Health Provider ____
Policy/Group Number ____
Authorization Phone ____

❐ I have advance directives (Living Will) attached ❐ I have no advance directives
❐ I use oxygen ❐ I am an organ donor ❐ I am an eye donor

MEDICATION	DOSAGE	WHY I TAKE IT	TIMES TAKEN	SIDE EFFECTS	SPECIAL INFO (Take with food, etc.)

School Asthma Plan

Name ____
Age and Grade ______________________________________
School ____
School Phone _______________________________________
Teacher ____

Contact Parent/Guardian If: ___________________________
____

Parent/Guardian Name ________________________________
Phones ____
If Parent/Guardian Unavailable, Contact _________________
Phones ____

Physician ____
Phone ____
Hospital Preference __________________________________

Allergies: Medications ________________________________
____

Allergies: Food ______________________________________
____

Allergies: Other _____________________________________
____

My Peak Flow Zones Are:
Green ____
Yellow ____
Red ____

My Medications Are: (Name, Dosage, When to Use) __________
____
____

Medications: ❒ Kept At School ❒ With Child ❒ Other __________
Activity Restrictions __________________________________
____

Teacher Signature and Date ____________________________

Parent Signature and Date _____________________________

Resources

Sneeze The Day!™ Newsletter – FREE SAMPLE OFFER

Everything you've read in this book first appeared in *Sneeze The Day!* For the latest news and information about living with your allergies, asthma or pulmonary condition, subscribe to *Sneeze The Day!* One year (6 issues) is $18, and major credit cards or a personal check are accepted. For a FREE SAMPLE ISSUE, call, write or e-mail, and mention the free sample offer in the Inspiration book.
1-800-968-1738
Good Communications, Inc.
PO Box 10069, Dept IN
Austin, TX 78766
E-mail: gooddogmag@aol.com
Fax: 512-454-3420

American Academy of Allergy and Immunology
611 East Wells Street
Milwaukee, WI 53202
(414) 272-6071

American Allergy Association
P.O.Box 7273
Menlo Park, CA 94025 - 7273
(415) 322-1663

American Association of Respiratory Care
11030 Abel Lane
Dallas, TX 75229-4524
(214) 243-2272

American College of Allergy and Immunology
800 E Northwest Highway, Suite 1080
Palatine, IL 60067-6516

American College of Chest Physicians
911 Busse Highway
Park Ridge, IL 6002
(708) 359-2800

American Lung Association
1740 Broadway
New York, NY 10019
(212) 315-8700
1-800-LUNG-USA

Hayfever Prevention Society
Rosewell Gardens Ste 2-G
2300 Sedgwick Ave.
Bronx, NY 10468
(212) 295-1069

The LAM Foundation
10105 Beacon Hills Drive
Cincinnati, OH 45241
(513) 777-6889

Mothers of Asthmatics, Inc.
10875 Main Street, Suite 210
Fairfax, VA 22030
(703) 385-4403

National Asthma Education Program
NHLBI Information Center
PO Box 30105
Bethesda, MD 20814-0105

National Heart, Lung and Blood Institute
9000 Rockville Pike
Bethesda, MD 20892
(301) 951-3260

National Immune Deficiency Foundation
Courthouse Square
3565 Ellicott Mills Drive, Unit B2
Ellicott City, MD 21043
1-800-296-4433

National Institute of Allergy and Infectious Diseases
Building 31, Room 7A32
Bethesda, MD 20892
(301) 496-5717

National Jewish Center for Immunology and Respiratory Medicine
1400 Jackson Street
Denver, CO 80206
(303) 388-4461

PRODUCTS

ALCAT Blood Test for Food and Other Sensitivities
American Medical Testing Laboratories
One Oakwood Blvd., Suite 130
Hollywood, FL 33020
1-800-881-AMTL

Aller-Caire
National distributor to consumers of top-quality, brand-name environmental products, including Cloud 9 HEPAs, Nilfisk and Eureka Europa vacuums, and Allergy Control Products encasements.
Aller-Caire
1617 Ogden Ave.
Lisle, IL 60532
1-800-547-8095

Dust Mite Control for Steam Cleaners
Ecology Works Dust Mite Control
415-488-0234

Priorities Allergy Products Catalog
70 Walnut Street
Wellesley, MA 02181-2175
1-800-553-5398

Whole House Dehumidifier for Dust Mite Control
Therma-Stor Products
1919 S Stoughton Rd., PO Box 8050
Madison, WI 53708
1-800-533-7533
www.thermastor.com